David Young

Rome in winter, and the Tuscan hills in summer : a contribution to the climate of Italy

David Young

Rome in winter, and the Tuscan hills in summer : a contribution to the climate of Italy

ISBN/EAN: 9783337229344

Printed in Europe, USA, Canada, Australia, Japan

Cover: Foto ©Andreas Hilbeck / pixelio.de

More available books at **www.hansebooks.com**

ROME IN WINTER

AND

THE TUSCAN HILLS IN SUMMER

A CONTRIBUTION TO THE CLIMATE OF ITALY

BY

DAVID YOUNG, M.C., M.B., M.D.

LICENTIATE OF THE ROYAL COLLEGE OF PHYSICIANS, EDINBURGH
LICENTIATE OF THE ROYAL COLLEGE OF SURGEONS, EDINBURGH
LATE PROFESSOR OF BOTANY IN THE GRANT MEDICAL COLLEGE, BOMBAY
FELLOW OF, AND LATE EXAMINER IN MIDWIFERY TO, THE UNIVERSITY OF BOMBAY
AND FELLOW OF THE OBSTETRICAL SOCIETY OF LONDON

LONDON
H. K. LEWIS, 136 GOWER STREET, W.C.
1886

TO

MY WIFE,

THE LOVED AND ONLY COMPANION OF MANY OF THE JOURNEYS
HEREIN DESCRIBED.

THE AUTHOR.

PREFACE.

No capital and indeed no city in Europe presents greater attractions to visitors from all lands than the city of the Seven Hills, and no city is more dreaded for its *supposed* unhealthiness.

The former none will question, and the latter may, by a calm consideration of the facts, presented in the following pages, be found to be largely due to ignorance, and the exaggerations of travellers. One fact must ever be borne in mind in forming conclusions as to the sanitary condition of Rome from the number of distinguished visitors who may have died there, and that is, that no continental city is visited by so many persons of distinction as Rome.

Savants of all nationalities drawn hither by its vast treasures in archæology, art, science and religion, crowd within its walls, and a death occurring amongst them naturally attracts attention in a wider circle than that of any ordinary and less well-known traveller.

Many deaths from typhoid fever occur in Paris, Berlin, Vienna and Dresden without attracting a tithe of the notice which *one* death does from the same cause in Rome, when occurring in the class of distinguished strangers, so many of whom frequent the city of the Cæsars.

The following chapters, written during the leisure of a brief summer holiday, show that Rome has not deserved the reputation which has so long attached to it for *unhealthiness*, and that it has suffered, not a little, from misrepresentations of its true sanitary condition. Excepting the treatise by Sir James Clark, written now many years ago, no book exists in our language which treats of Rome and its climate. The present volume is an attempt to supply this want.

The principal elements in the climate are briefly described—the prevailing diseases are compared with those of England and northern countries generally, and the *type* of diseases likely to receive benefit in Italy is dwelt on at some length, while the sanitary state of the city and the important and increasingly interesting subject of Malaria are also considered. One or two of the chapters appeared in *The Practitioner* a few years ago, but have been rewritten and modified as further experience has rendered necessary.

To *The Lancet* and *The British Medical Journal*, as well as to the various authorities mentioned in the text, I desire to express my obligations for the assistance which I have derived from them.

DAVID YOUNG, M.D.

ROME, *December*, 1885.

TABLE OF CONTENTS.

CHAP.
I.—SOME REMARKS ON CLIMATES GENERALLY AND THEIR EFFECTS ON MORBID CONDITIONS.

II.—THE CLIMATE OF ROME AND ITS EFFECTS UPON HEALTH AND DISEASE.

III.—THE UNHEALTHINESS OF ROME.

IV.—ROMAN FEVER AND MALARIA.

V.—THE WATER SUPPLY OF ROME.

VI.—HOW TO LIVE IN ROME.

VII.—SUMMER QUARTERS NEAR ROME.

VIII.—SUMMER QUARTERS IN TUSCANY.

IX.—THE CLASS OF INVALIDS LIKELY TO DERIVE BENEFIT FROM A RESIDENCE IN ROME.

CONTENTS.

CHAPTER I.

Effects of Season upon Health—Treatment of Phthisis by means of Climate—Sea and Mountain Climates—A Sea Voyage—Air on Board Steam Ships—Moist and Dry Air—Climate and Scrofula—Physical properties of the Atmosphere—High Altitudes—Observations at the Abetone—Floating Matters in the Air—Bacteria—Absolute and relative Moisture—Coldness of Mountain Air—Formation of Dew—Fogs and Mists—Ozone—Goitre and Malaria—Eucalyptus trees . . 1

CHAPTER II.

Configuration of the Coast of Italy—The Mediterranean—The City of Rome—The Campagna—Rome as a Winter Residence—Annual Mean Temperature—Rainfall—Prevailing Winds—Ozone—Prevailing Diseases in England and Italy—Malarial Cases in Male and Female Hospitals in Rome—Diphtheria and Croup—Proportion of Acute to Chronic Diseases in Italy—Degenerative Changes 42

CHAPTER III.

The Unhealthiness of Rome—Typhoid in Rome and Paris—A Death in Dresden—Sanitary Condition of Rome—Roman Churches and their Burying Grounds—Pernicious Influence of Stagnant Pools—Modern Closets—*A Sanitary Festa*—Malarial Fever—Unhealthy Dwellings—The Jews in the Ghetto—*Febbre Perniciosa*—Diphtheria and Small-pox—Deaths from Typhoid in Italy and London—Number of English and American Visitors in Rome—Roman Wells . 70

CHAPTER IV.

Roman Fever—Subcontinued Typhoid—Experience of Roman Fever in Florence—Quinine in Roman Fever—Cases of Roman Fever—Experience in Rome—Infective Malaria—True Nature of Roman Fever—The Roman Campagna—Nature of Malaria—Malaria at Sea—A Damp Bedroom—Bacillus Malariæ—Modes of Entrance into Human Body—Life History of Malarial Parasite—Effects of Water upon—Conveyed by Water 101

CHAPTER V.

Water Supply—Early Roman Engineers—Settling Reservoirs—Curatores Aquarum—Aqua Marcia—Aqua Tepula and Julia—Aqua di Trevi—Aqua Paola and Felice—Pollution of Aqua di Trevi—Source of Aqua di Trevi—Disease Germs in Water—Organic Matters in Water—Oxygen Method—Mineral Constituents of Roman Waters—Common Salt in Trevi Water—Trevi Water at Source and in Rome—Probable Causes of Pollution—Sources of Aqua Marcia—Receiving Chamber of Aqua Marcia 152

CHAPTER VI.

Precautions to be taken in Rome—Chief Dangers of Roman Climate—Cold Weather in Rome—Choice of an Apartment—Roman Habits—Acclimatization—Warm Clothing—Imprudences of Visitors—Animal Food—Sleeplessness—Sightseeing—Exposure at Sunset 189

CHAPTER VII.

Mineral Waters in Italy—Alban and Sabine Towns—Seaside Resorts—Civita Vecchia—Palo—Porto D'Anzio—Tivoli—Subiaco—Olevano—Albano—Frascati—Rocca di Papa—Monte Cavo 201

CHAPTER VIII.

Montecatini and Monsummano—La Spezia—Vallombrosa—Camaldoli—Prato Vecchio—Sacro Eremo—Alvernia—Bagni di Lucca—The Mountains of Pistoia—Gavinana—San Marcello—Cutigliano—The Abetone—Road to Abetone—The Forest of Abetone—Climate of Abetone—Hotels and Pensions at Abetone—Certosa di Pesio—Andorno . . 218

CHAPTER IX.

Influence of the Mediterranean—Effects of Italian Climate upon Chronic Disease—Earliest Symptoms of Broken Health—Importance of these Early Symptoms—Description of Early Symptoms—More Advanced Symptoms—Personal Experiences—Cases Suitable for Rome—Holiday for Professional Men—Cases Unsuitable for Rome—Abuse of Quinine . 259

WINTER IN ITALY.

CHAPTER I.

Effects of Season upon Health—Treatment of Phthisis by means of Climate—Sea and Mountain Climates—A Sea Voyage—Air on Board Steam Ships—Moist and Dry Air—Climate and Scrofula—Physical properties of the Atmosphere—High Altitudes—Observations at the Abetone—Floating Matters in the Air—Bacteria—Absolute and relative Moisture—Coldness of Mountain Air—Formation of Dew—Fogs and Mists—Ozone—Goitre and Malaria—Eucalyptus trees.

MORE than twenty years ago, one of the most accomplished, thoughtful, and successful physicians in the Scottish capital gave the following advice to a young practitioner about to set out on his medical career: "Observe carefully the effects of weather upon your patients, watch closely how Nature helps them by air and sunshine, and you will soon discover that, under many circumstances, *change of air* is one of the most potent remedies in the cure of disease." The advice was sound, but the subject was not by any means new, nor even of modern origin. Many of the fathers of medicine would have said the same thing. Hippocrates wrote, "The maladies engendered by winter, cease in the summer; those engendered by summer, cease in the winter. The cure of disorders engendered by spring may be expected in the autumn; that of maladies engendered by the autumn must necessarily take place in the spring."

The effects of season upon health are, moreover, matters known to every one, and of daily observation. The east wind in England, and the Tramontana in Italy, have acquired a just notoriety for the evil effects which they exert upon health and disease, and count annually vast numbers who succumb to their influence. Indeed, the Tramontana in Italy is far more to be dreaded by visitors than the malaria, about which so much has been said and written in recent years. The experience of the effects of season and weather both in aiding and retarding recovery from illness, as well as their influence upon the healthy organism, is not confined to the few or to any class of society in particular.

Is it not, then, somewhat remarkable that a subject which attracted attention in bygone ages, which has been making itself felt, with such constancy and so much force, from the days when the members of the healing art professed to receive their inspiration from the planets down to our own time, should have made so little real advance? There must be a reason why there is not a greater consensus of opinion among medical men in a branch of medical science at once so interesting in itself, and capable of producing such important results. The reason is not to be found in any paucity in the number of observers, or in the amount of work which has been accomplished. A great deal of work of a kind has been done, and meteorological and other observations have been accumulating for a lengthened period in various parts of the world. Of late years, also, the rapid growth of so-called health resorts, and the remarkable advance which has recently taken place in the treatment of certain forms of pulmonary disease by a residence in cold, dry, mountain districts, have brought many new facts to light, and considerably enriched our knowledge of medical climatology; and yet, when we come to examine the literature of the subject as a purely medical inquiry, we find it very meagre, and very few are the statistics which we meet with which throw much light upon the *modus operandi* of climate upon disease, or, in other words, the manner in which changes of climate affect the human body in health and disease. A medical friend who has long practised on the Riviera, tells me that among his phthisical patients, attacks of hæmoptysis will occur, affecting several persons at the same time, and leaving no doubt upon his mind that changes in the weather preceding the attacks were the exciting causes. Nor should this be a matter of surprise, as any one conversant with the physical condition of the lungs, especially in certain stages of pulmonary consumption, will readily see that a sudden fall of temperature may lead, in these cases, to congestion of some portion of the diseased organs and so become a cause of hæmorrhage. From a few and imperfect observations which the writer made at the Abetone, some years ago, he found that cold, damp weather coming on suddenly after a period of warm sunshine, invariably increased the discomfort and difficulty of breathing in the case of three patients suffering from phthisis who were under his care during the whole of the summer. Auscultation at these times revealed increased hyperæmia of the affected lungs—the cough was drier and more difficult—and musical ronchi were heard where previously they did not exist.

The treatment of phthisis by means of climate—the most advanced outpost of medical climatology—

must, however, still be regarded as in its infancy, if we take into consideration the great variety of climates recommended by physicians for their patients, a variety so great as to include places having atmospheric conditions the opposite of one another. Some patients are sent to seaside resorts where the air is warm and moist, others far inland where it is warm and dry, some again are advised to go to low Alpine places, having an air which is cold as well as damp, and others to great Alpine heights such as Davos, St. Moritz, the Maloja, Quito and La Paz, where it is cold and dry; while yet another class—perhaps the largest class of all—are told to set their house in order and, whether they are good sailors or bad, advised for a time to make their home upon the ocean. It has long been said and believed that "doctors differ," and the recent attempts which have been made to revive the *climatic theory* of disease, so well understood by Hippocrates, have neither lessened the frequency of the saying nor the belief that it is true. If a change of residence on account of illness has to be made, it is the most reasonable and natural thing in the world for the patient to desire to know what it is he is avoiding, and what it is he is to find in the new home which he is exchanging for the old one. This desire on the part of the patient, or his relatives, is not only reasonable, but it is pre-eminently just. It is, however, a desire not so easy to gratify; and though we possess so little knowledge of the etiological and therapeutic influence of meteorological phenomena, yet we invariably act as if we had a most intimate knowledge of the subject. Two reasons are readily found to explain this apparent anomaly. There are many cases of consumption, as well as of other affections, which derive benefit from a given climate; but the same amount of good has also been found to accrue in the same class of cases, when under the influence of another climate presenting widely different physical characteristics from the former; hence it is that patients suffering from pulmonary phthisis, or having phthisical tendencies, have derived incalcuable benefit by a residence at Davos or Quito; while others have been rescued from the grasp of their enemy by a prolonged sea voyage. When comparing sea with mountain climates, later on, I hope to be able to show that this experience is in strict accordance with what might be expected from recent scientific discoveries. But there is a second reason which partly accounts for the diversity of opinion which prevails, and that is that we are not sufficiently acquainted with the forces which are at work exerting their influence upon disease in such a manner as to lead to beneficial results in one climate, while they cause the patient to lose ground in another. In a recent voyage which I made from Naples to London in one of the comfortable steamers belonging to the Orient Line, I had an opportunity of seeing several phthisical patients who were returning from Australia after a residence in the Colony, or who were simply making the trip *out* and *home*. Some were bronzed, had gained flesh and strength, had lost their cough and spoke hopefully of the future; while others had gradually become feebler and weaker, and were longing to reach their homes again. One of these latter cases interested me very deeply. It was that of a young gentleman, aged twenty-eight, who had caught cold while out shooting on the moors; the attack proved to be one of double pneumonia, from which he was thought to have made a good recovery; but a certain delicacy of chest was left, and towards the end of the summer a voyage to Australia was recommended, and now he was returning home in the last stage of pulmonary phthisis. The attentions of the doctor enabled him to live on till the ship reached Gravesend, where his young wife met him and took him ashore. So little was such a result expected that she was advised not to accompany him, and the strongest hopes were held out that he would probably return without a trace of lung weakness about him.

What valuable contributions to medical climatology would carefully made clinical observations be in cases like this. Placed under climatic conditions apparently so favourable, what were the causes which led to such an unlooked for issue? All we really know is, that this patient was advised to make a voyage to Australia in order to secure the beneficial effects of climate in one of its purest forms by a prolonged residence upon the ocean, with the disappointing result that he returned to England immeasurably worse than when he left. Probably the hygienic conditions under which he made the voyage may have had some influence in bringing about such an unexpected termination. The air on the open sea is the purest of all climates, but the same thing cannot be always said of the air on board steam ships; and we must not shut our eyes to the fact that wherever a large number of people congregate, and especially if there are several consumptive invalids among them, the air may be found to be very impure.

It was reported among the passengers that during this voyage there had been one case of mild typhoid, and one or two of scarlet fever, as well as several cases of troublesome sore throat.

These reports did not surprise me, for, notwithstanding that the ship was visited almost daily by the captain in company with the doctor, the sanitary state of the cabinets used by the first class passengers was anything but good, more especially in stormy weather. While the portions of the vessel occupied by the second and third class passengers suggested even greater dangers. Much of all this is necessarily inseparable from life at sea, and should be borne in mind in all cases where a sea voyage is advised.

To these may also be added the confusion which prevails owing to the want of precision which obtains in the terms employed to express some of the ordinary conditions of the atmosphere; cold and warm, severe and mild, moist and dry are used relatively, and may be used by different persons with reference to weather of the same place and at the same time, and this is true of physicians as well as of patients. A medical writer on climate in London speaking of Madeira, describes it as *warm and moist*, while several other medical men well acquainted with the island from residence in it, say it is *warm and dry*. A more important practical point for discussion would have been, What are its effects upon the organism, what morbid processes does it seem to promote, and what are the others it is likely to hinder? Moreover, such contention to have Madeira placed among dry rather than amongst moist climates gives the impression that the moisture in its air is something to be dreaded. There appears to be a very widespread notion that such really is the case, and no element in the physical properties of the atmosphere has been more soundly abused than its watery vapour, and yet, how much in our day are some lung and throat affections treated by means of *saturated air* in the form of medicated and simple steam inhalations. Another well known author, writing of Davos to the *Lancet* says, "the difference between the wet and dry bulbs was only 2·8° Fahr., showing how *great* the *dryness* of the air is." According to the ordinary method of estimating the humidity of the air by the difference between the wet and dry bulbs a difference of only 2·8° Fahr. would rather indicate that the climate was *not very dry*. In a little *brochure* commending a favourite Scotch spa situated about 200 feet above the level of the sea, the practising physician describes the air of the place "as being much the same as the air of the Engadine"! When we remember the respective altitudes of the two places, the one being scarcely 200 *feet* and the other over 6,000 *feet* above the sea, it is evident that we have much to attain to in the matter of precision in the language we use.

In studying climate from a medical point of view it is essential to be borne in mind that the influence of external causes upon the constitution of living creatures is very great and varies with locality. That these causes, moreover, are not only very numerous in themselves, but also an endless variety of results is produced by them according to their combination, while there are what may be termed compensatory arrangements in the organism itself, which to some extent—probably to a greater extent than we know—counteract and modify these climatic influences. But further, there are certain compensatory laws which exist among the physical forces themselves, and exert a considerable influence upon the action which they would naturally exercise upon the living body. A familiar example of this is seen in warm climates having a high degree of *absolute* moisture. The more aqueous vapour in the atmosphere the greater is its power of *conducting* warmth, and therefore the more will it help organic bodies to part with their heat. It does this, however, under certain circumstances, only to a limited extent. Generally speaking, the effects of high temperature upon the human body are to cause a greater functional activity of the skin, producing an increasing perspiration; but the greater amount of *relative* moisture in these climates tends to check the evaporation of perspiration, and so lessen the great heat loss from the body which an otherwise absolutely moist air would cause. In endeavouring, therefore, to ascertain the effects of weather upon morbid processes we must not forget to take these influences into account. Neither must we fail to remember that there are others, apparently trifling and imponderable in themselves, which are as yet only partially known and appreciated, but which influence, in no small degree, the results of attempts made to obtain from the various climates of the world their healing effects for ourselves and our suffering fellow men. It is not therefore *opinions* but *facts* that we require to guide us in our further search, and if the many earnest workers in all lands would devote themselves to a closer observation of the varying changes of weather in the relation they bear to the varying changes in disease, thus establishing the correlation of weather and disease, a greater consensus of opinion would exist amongst medical men, and we would, ere long, be in a better position to answer the question so often anxiously put to us: " Will a change of climate have any effect in arresting the progress of the malady?" A question which has so frequently made us sensible of our ignorance of the principles which alone should guide us in our endeavour to give a satisfactory answer to it. It will be readily seen from what has been said, that purely meteorological facts in themselves are of little value in elucidating the intricate subject before us, and that because in England certain climatic conditions, such as dampness or coldness of the air, appear to have a retarding influence upon the recovery from certain diseased conditions, we are to assume that exactly the same results will accrue under similar atmospheric conditions in a different latitude. A much more hopeful field—as in speaking of Italy I may be able to show—seems to present itself in the observation of prevailing diseases under tolerably similar conditions of the air, but in different latitudes, and also in dissimilar atmospheric conditions whether in the same or in other latitudes.

The venerable Dr. Gutike made a number of very valuable observations on this point in Germany, and speaking of Halle and Magdeburg, he says that "the scrofulous tendency in young persons is removed if they are sent from Halle to Magdeburg or from Magdeburg to Halle, and yet both of these towns are similar as regards climate; they are both the same height above the sea, and the soil in the one place very much resembles the soil in the other." But what is still more startling is, " both are equally notorious seats of scrofula, and both places have alike suffered from severe epidemics of the disease." Thousands of consumptive patients have been sent to Australia, and a large proportion have derived very great benefit from going there ; while not a few similar cases have come to England from Australia, and have likewise reaped decided good from the change.

In some functional disturbances of the uterus which have come under my notice, residence in London has been the apparent cause, and Brighton has been credited with their removal ; while the same kind of derangements occurring in Brighton have completely disappeared after a brief stay in London, and this without any medical treatment whatever. Florence is well known for its influence as a cause of amenorrhœa in young healthy English girls, while as far as my experience goes, the opposite condition is produced by the climate of Rome; and it is now a generally received fact that consumptive patients should never be sent to Ems, as the number of cases of hæmoptysis occurring in that deservedly popular and important Spa, prove it to be dangerous for them.

All this warns us not to be too ready in accepting physical theories, and that much more is required than mere meteorological tables to establish a relation between health resorts enjoying similar climatic characteristics and geographical position, as well as not to believe it impossible that like results may be obtained at places very dissimilar in point of climate as well as geographical position.

The attention of the observer should be directed more especially to the following features in the climate, while at the same time, prevailing diseases and marked variations in their course, attributed to climatic influences, should also be recorded.

The temperature and barometric pressure of the air, and its freedom from microbes.

Humidity.

Winds, and presence of ozone.

It may seem somewhat strange that notwithstanding the great increase which has been made in our knowledge of the modes and causes of phthisis in recent years, very little has been gained for our guidance as to the part which variations in temperature and barometric pressure play in producing the beneficial results which have been recorded since consumption began to be treated by what may be termed *climatic treatment;* and this, too, in spite of the fact that until quite recently the attention of observers was attracted to meteorological phenomena almost exclusively. In those results which have been obtained in cases of pulmonary phthisis, there is now an almost universal unanimity of opinion that the *purity* of the air, that is, its freedom from germs, is the main factor in their production; and that while the nature of the soil and geological formation have no mean claims to be regarded as agents in conferring the comparative immunity from this disease, which some districts enjoy more than others; yet it is a fact, that both the temperature and pressure of the air, apart from other considerations, exert considerable influence over the processes of repair in diseased tissues, and offer a hopeful practical ground upon which we can to some extent rely in seeking to determine the question as to whether a given case might derive greater benefit by a change to the seaside than to the mountains, or *vice versâ*. The physical properties of the atmosphere at the sea-side, and in high altitudes, present several striking contrasts, as well as several no less important similarities; and in connection with these properties, involving the quantities of oxygen and ozone, the temperature, sunlight, movements and pressure of the air, as well as its freedom from microbes, we have a natural basis for arranging all climates under three practical heads. These are as follows:—

1. Warm sea climates.
2. Cold dry mountain climates.
3. Warm inland climates.

The chief characteristics of sea-climates are

1. Greater density of the air.
2. Abundance of ozone.
3. Abundance of moisture.
4. Freedom from dust of all kinds.
5. Equability of temperature.
6. Barometric oscillations considerable, but regular.
7. More or less constant movement of the air by land and sea breezes, as well as by more distant winds.
8. Intensity of light.
9. Presence of some saline matters and a small quantity of bromine and iodine.

The main features of mountain climates are

1. Diminished pressure.
2. Cool, or even cold.
3. Abundance of ozone.
4. Absence of moisture.
5. Freedom from dust.

6. Calm in winter, and *windy* in summer.

7. Warmer sunshine than at low levels.

The physiological effects of marine and mountain climates upon the diseased as well as upon the healthy individual, present some important contrasts. At the sea-side there is greater heat loss, and therefore greater activity in change of tissue, so that nutritive changes are less active in the mountains than by the sea, and greater care is necessary to prevent the body being chilled at the sea than in higher altitudes—the temperature being the same. Professor Beneke of Marburg, who has made some very interesting observations on this subject, further states that, with the increased activity of oxidation, as seen by the excess of urea and sulphuric acid, there is diminution of phosphoric and uric acids, and increase of body-weight. This is an important advance in our knowledge.

In a large class of cases of disease, the great desideratum is to promote nutritive changes in the body, thus favouring the throwing off of old material and the building up with new. The favourable results obtained in cases of pulmonary disease by marine climates would appear, therefore, to be due to the presence in large quantity of oxygen and ozone, promoting the changes due to active oxidation, and at the same time exerting a destructive influence upon the existence of the bacilli of the lung, a function which is promoted by the powerful antiseptic properties of the bromine and iodine, with their combinations.

The effects produced by a residence in high altitudes, as at St. Moritz and Davos, are at the outset increased action of the heart both as to energy and frequency of beat, while the respirations are quicker. After a time both heart and lungs accommodate themselves to the rarefied atmosphere and act somewhat more slowly. The amount of oxygen consumed is much less than at the sea-side, while the elimination of carbonic acid and of water by the *lungs* is greatly increased, owing to the extreme coldness and dryness of the air. The results obtained in cases of phthisis at these high elevations compare favourably with those already mentioned as occurring at the sea. An examination of the chief factors in producing these results will readily show why such similar results should accrue from climates *apparently* so diverse in physical properties and physiological effects. The conditions which are common to both are purity of air, freedom from germs, and abundance of ozone; the two great points of contrast being that while the one contains bromine and iodine, the other is cold instead of being warm, and as rarefaction is characteristic of mountain air, so density is one of the main features of sea air. While, therefore, active oxidation is carried on at the sea-side owing to the denser air with more oxygen and ozone, the same process is maintained at high altitudes with less oxygen but increased frequency in the number of respirations, the diminution of pressure facilitating the complete aëration of the lungs and so preventing the bacilli from multiplying. The disinfecting power of the bromine and iodine is more than compensated for by the extreme coldness and dryness of mountain air, which have a deleterious effect upon bacilli and other microbes, rendering them innocuous. Keeping in mind these relations between marine and mountain climates, and observing the variations in disease in different localities, we may be able to decide with greater precision what cases are more suitable for the one climate than for the other.

It is not enough to say that any particular case of phthisis or some other disease has been " arrested," or "improved," or "much improved ;" we want to know more than this, and if possible find out what the weather has to say to it, and what changes in the temperature and pressure of the air influence the malady, and whether, by knowing these, we cannot promote recovery from certain diseased conditions by placing the patient under more favourable circumstances in regard to climate and weather. A few years ago, during a summer spent at The Abetone, I made the observations already referred to on this subject, and was both interested and surprised to find that on days when the air contained a large amount of ozone several patients with bronchial and laryngeal affections complained of increased irritation and a greater tendency to cough, while three persons suffering from phthisis, all in advanced stages of the disease, apparently suffered less than the others, and, indeed, complained very little. On the other hand, during cold damp weather, the case was reversed, and the former patients suffered little or no inconvenience, whereas the latter became more restless, feverish, and irritable, and auscultation revealed evidence of increased hyperæmia of the lungs in the shape of clear musical ronchi in the neighbourhood of condensations and cavities where they were not heard before. Two cases of chronic rheumatism, with deposits in the joints, were not so much affected on damp days as I had expected, and when they did suffer from painful stiffness in the joints and other discomforts I was not able at first to trace anything remarkable in the weather either as to cold or dampness to account for it; but glancing over my meteorological tables I invariably found that these days were notably colder than the days which had preceded them, and though less cold and less damp than many which we had experienced they seemed to influence these cases to a greater degree, and I could only account for it by supposing that it was more owing to the *sudden change* from warm dry weather to cold damp weather than either the degree of coldness or dampness in itself. A young lady with lateral curvature of the spine, very anæmic and with a family history of phthisis, found dry cold weather suit her better than damp weather. On cold damp days she nearly always complained of shooting pains through her chest, and invariably suffered from diarrhœa; while an old Indian recently returned from India and suffering from enlarged liver and spleen, with constipation, flatulence, and acidity after eating, experienced an exaggeration of all his symptoms in cold dry weather, while he was comparatively comfortable on days which were moister, even though they were also cold. Few in number and imperfect as these observations are they are of little value, and are only referred to as suggestive and indicating the kind of observations which are necessary to the elucidation of many points which are still very obscure in the relations which exist between weather and disease, and more particularly between variations in the weather and changes occurring during the progress of disease.

Regarding the purity of the air, recent years have made us acquainted with many new facts illustrative of the dangers which surround us in the atmosphere, laden as it is with the seeds of disease which at this moment are attracting such universal attention. Formerly, investigations into the purity of the atmosphere were mainly directed to its physical composition, which is subject to very little variations in the mountains, on the plains, or by the seashore ; but since the facts brought to light by Pasteur, Tyndall and Lister, the attention of medical climatologists has been directed to a new aspect of the question in the shape of floating matters in the air. These floating matters, or dust particles, are derived from organic as well as from inorganic sources, and to the former a comparatively greater degree of importance is attachable than to the latter.

Organic dust particles appear to the naked eye as *motes* in sunbeams, and in bad or impure air in the neglected and unhealthy parts of large cities where human beings crowd together these germs are found in such quantities as to be sensible both to smell and taste ; while a large portion of these germs is so invisible as to be beyond the power of any microscope to detect, and their presence is only declared when the air containing them is illumined by the sunbeam or the beam of the electric light, when a peculiar opalescence becomes visible, due to these ultramicroscopic microbes. Many of these minute organisms are now well-known, and besides playing a very important part in the causation of disease, they likewise fulfil many other functions not only invaluable, but even necessary to life. These minute living bodies have proved in the hands of Pasteur the means of saving multitudes of sheep and cattle from death by anthrax, they are the essential agents in the digestion of our food, they make our bread and turn our grapes into wine, without them our crops would not grow, and much of our dairy produce would be valueless. This teeming world of microscopic life thus contains innumerable agents of minutest form, highly serviceable to man, and others which are equally hurtful and even fatal to him. Could we discover the means of destroying the latter, mildew and blight would disappear from our fields, our potatoes and grapes would be preserved to us, while such diseases as typhoid fever, scarlatina, diphtheria, erysipelas and measles would be unknown.

Numerous experiments have been conducted with the view of ascertaining the amount of these floating microbes in the air of dwellings, in cities, on mountain tops and upon the sea, and M. Miguel of the Observatoire de Montsouris, near Paris, whose researches are deeply interesting and of the highest value, gives the following table as the result of his experiments:—

	Bacteria, per 10 Cub. Metres.
1. Elevation of from 2,000 to 4,000 metres	None
2. On the Lake of Thun, 560 metres	8·0
3. Near the Hotel Bellevue, Thun, 560 metres	25·0
4. In a room of the Hotel Bellevue	600·0
5. In the park of Montsouris, Paris	7,600·0
6. In Paris. Rue de Rivoli	35,000·0

From this table one reason will be readily seen why it is that consumptive patients have fared so well in Alpine climates; and from some experiments which have been conducted at sea, although on a very small scale, there is reason to believe that sea climates have an equal immunity from bacterial germs where there is no contamination by the proximity of large cities. The existence of these active agents in the atmosphere gives additional importance to medical climatology, and until we know how to destroy them, our next care must be to place susceptible patients beyond their reach.

The humidity of the atmosphere is, next to its purity, perhaps the most important physical condition. According to their degree of humidity, climates have been divided into moist and dry, but this division is a purely arbitrary one, and has no definite signification whatever.

The influence of the moisture of the air upon the human body is of very great practical importance, especially in certain conditions of disease. To obtain a tolerably clear understanding of the somewhat intricate subject of atmospheric humidity it will be necessary to refer to the causes which regulate the amount of moisture in the air, as all atmospheres do not contain the same amount of aqueous vapour, neither are they capable of doing so.

Two states of the atmosphere regulate its capacity for containing water,—these states are temperature and density. Vapour always rises up into the air from water by evaporation, but the evaporating power of an atmosphere is very different according as the air temperature is 32° or 60°. When, therefore, evaporation is going on from any surface, the minute particles of water which ascend into the air are invisible, and float about in the interspaces between the atoms of oxygen and nitrogen. They are so very minute, and they are separated so far from each other that they are invisible, and therefore water in this thinly-spread-out condition may be compared to a gas. The atmosphere can only hold a certain amount of these minute watery molecules to fill up the interspaces between its own atoms of oxygen and nitrogen, but a cold air can receive much less than a warm one, and the degree of capacity increases much faster than the rise in the thermometer. An atmosphere which has received all the water it is capable of holding in the invisible state is said to be saturated, and when in this condition the slightest diminution of temperature would cause the invisible vapour to become mist,—the watery molecules crowd together to form water, which falls through the air as fine rain. The amount of vapour which can be stowed away by the air in the interspaces between its own atoms has been accurately calculated. Thus a given volume of air at 32° Fahr. can sustain only $\frac{1}{160}$ part of its own weight of transparent vapour, while at 80° Fahr. it will hold nearly $\frac{1}{40}$th of its weight. The weight of the watery vapour in every cubic foot of saturated air at 32° Fahr. is 2·27 grains, at 60° Fahr. is 5·87 grs., and at 80 Fahr. 10·81 grs., and so therefore if the latter atmosphere was cooled down to 60° Fahr suddenly, it would part with its moisture to the extent of nearly 5 grains of rain out of each cubic foot. This is indeed one of the great functions of the atmosphere. It draws up vapours from both sea and land, retains them in itself in invisible forms or suspended in the clouds, and returns them to the earth again as dew, or rain, or snow. Warm air stores up the invisible vapour, floats it away on the wings of the wind, and then, reaching a cooler climate, throws it down as drops of rain. This evaporation which is always going on whatever be the temperature of the air, is increased somewhat by low barometric pressure, and also by winds which favour the dispersion of the moisture as it ascends. To express the humidity of the air two terms are usually employed, viz., Absolute moisture and Relative moisture. The distinction of the two is a matter of importance as the effects of the one upon the living organism are not the same as those produced by the other. By the term Absolute moisture is meant the amount of aqueous vapour contained in a given volume of air; and by Relative moisture is meant the proportion which exists between the actual amount of water in the air, and the amount which would be required to saturate the air at a given temperature. Generally speaking, in temperate climates the absolute moisture of the atmosphere is greater in summer than in winter, owing to the greater capacity which warm air has for containing moisture, whereas the relative moisture is higher in winter than in summer, because the atmosphere is then nearly always saturated, and requires very little aqueous vapour to enable it to reach that point.

From a careful examination of a large number of statistics which I recently made, I found that the results upon the death rate of a given population during wet weather, as calculated by the number of rainy days, or the rainfall in inches, was in many instances not the same as when based upon the average *relative humidity*. Clinical experience shows that the influence of absolute moisture relates exclusively to the respiratory organs, and hence the frequency with which steam inhalations are now prescribed in laryngeal, bronchial, and other chest affections. Relative moisture on the other hand manifests its action upon the skin. In some cases, however, the effects of a high degree of absolute moisture, which might prove hurtful to living beings, is counteracted by the opposite effects of the relative moisture; a familiar example of which is seen in the warm and moist climates of the tropics. And it is instructive to observe that it is during the winter, when the amount of absolute moisture is less than in the summer, that there is a greater loss of moisture from the lungs, whereas in the summer time when the degree of relative moisture is less than in winter more water is lost by the skin. In considering the effects of mountain air upon phthisis it is not unreasonable to suppose that this watery loss from the lungs may have had some influence in producing the good results which have been obtained. From the few observations made at The Abetone some years ago, and already referred to, indications were given that while consumptive patients suffered during cold and damp weather, they felt comparatively well when the air was cold and dry. The phthisical resorts of Davos and St. Moritz are especially characterised by the dryness of their climate in winter, and even in seaside winter climates as well as those of low-lying inland plains, apart from temperature, as far as I have been able to gather statistics, they invariably show that when the element of dryness is *marked*, the results in certain stages of the disease are more favourable than when the air is moist, hence the beautiful resorts on the Riviera, as well as the desert climate along the Nile, have long enjoyed a deserved reputation in these cases.

Another important feature in regard to relative moisture is, that where it is comparatively high, the temperature is more equable and less subject to changes. This is easily accounted for. Professor Tyndall has shown that the rays of the sun passing through pure dry air scarcely impart any heat to it, and thus it is that on ascending high mountains the air gets continually colder and colder the higher we climb, even though the sun be scorchingly hot.

The reason is that though the sun's rays be hot, the air itself is cold, and therefore the main cause of the coldness of mountain climates is not due to the absence of the sun, but to the absence of warm ground, which is the great source of the heat communicated to the air. The sun's warmth is first given to the ground, and the cool air touching the warm ground becomes heated and carries away the heat it receives into the higher regions. Moist air, however, behaves in a different way, and arrests the rays of the sun and prevents them from reaching the ground, and not only does it thus act as a screen in preventing the sun from warming the earth, but it also acts in a similar manner in preventing the earth from parting with what heat it has already obtained, and therefore the clearer the night the colder is it likely to be. It is the clearness and dryness of the air of Italy, that cause such a difference in the temperature between day and night.

Closely related to the moisture of the air, and important in a medical aspect, is the formation of dew. During the day, and under the influence of the sun, there is constant evaporation going on while the earth, and through it the lower stratum of the air, are receiving heat from its rays. After sunset both the earth and the air yield up the heat which they have been accumulating during the warm hours of the day, and it radiates into space. The earth loses its heat quicker than the air, and the moisture which is in the stratum of air lying immediately above the ground becomes deposited on its cooled surface as dew. A familiar example of the manner in which dew is formed is seen when a crystal bottle filled with very cold water is brought into a warm room. Immediately the outside of the bottle becomes bedewed with moisture, and the simple explanation is that the warm air of the room contained a certain quantity of moisture in the thin, spread-out, invisible form, but the instant the warm air came in contact with the cold surface of the water bottle, its moisture, till now invisible, was thrown down as water. Dew is only deposited upon the surface of a body, when that body is cooler than the air in contact with it, and bright clear weather without wind is more favourable to its deposition than cloudy weather. It is frequently observed in the early morning that the turf along the sides of a road is covered with dew when the road itself is comparatively dry. The reason is that plants part with their heat more readily than rock or sand, and receive it more slowly; they are more easily cooled, and then their leaves become free surfaces for the condensation of the moisture in the air around them. This process of condensation is constantly going on in the atmosphere in the formation of mists and fogs, which are caused by the watery vapour depositing itself upon solid particles floating in the air. The dense yellow fogs of London and other great cities are partly due to the large amount of sulphur found in English coal, as well as to the admixture of smoke. These dense smoky fogs find their way even into dwelling-houses: whereas the pure white mists and fogs in country districts never do, as they are immediately dissipated by a slight degree of warmth.

The influence of wind as a factor in medical climatology has attracted considerable attention in all ages, and in our own time the endeavour has been made to establish a direct relationship between disease and mortality, and the prevalence of winds blowing in a particular direction.

It has been noted that all winds from a point between N. and E. indicate a direct relationship between their prevalence and disease and mortality. While on the other hand an inverse relationship is indicated between mortality and winds from a point between S. and W. All winds blowing from a point between N.W. and S.E. were found to attend a high death rate, while winds blowing from a point between S.E. and W. occurred more frequently when the death rate was low.

In the treatment of phthisis, the great desideratum has been to find a climate having cold, dry, pure air with absence of wind, and this has been found at Davos and other high mountain resorts.

The influence of stillness of atmosphere in very cold climates is of the highest value in enabling the body to support very great degrees of cold.

When an atmosphere is both dry and calm, an almost incredible degree of cold can be borne with impunity. In Siberia and in Canada, with the thermometer marking 40° Fahr. below zero, the air may be felt less cold than it is in a damp climate like England, when the thermometer is only a few degrees below freezing. A warm dry wind raises the temperature of the air and increases its capacity for moisture, thereby promoting evaporation, which has been found to be very much greater in windy than in still weather; while a cold wind lowers the temperature, and causes moisture to fall as dew, rain, or snow. The influence of the wind upon the human body is in proportion to its warmth, dryness, and force. It is said that during the prevalence of the dry Harmattan wind old ulcers cease to discharge; and it accords with my own experience that during the Tramontana scrofulous sores along the shores of the Mediterranean make more satisfactory progress than at other times. The only remaining element to be noticed is the presence of ozone in the air, and while much has been written about it, we are still too much in the dark, not only as to its nature, but even as to reliable methods for determining the quantity in the atmosphere to be able to say much as to the part it plays in medical climatology.

Before, therefore, we can hope to define its physiological action we must first know more about its chemistry. It is believed to be oxygen in an altered or allotropic condition, and is represented by O_2O; while antozone is supposed to be peroxide of hydrogen.

As an air purifier there is little doubt that ozone plays an important part, and much of the oxidation of the products of animal and vegetable waste, and their consequent removal from the air, may be performed by it. Attempts have been made to purify sick rooms by it, and in America an apparatus for producing ozone from the slow combustion of phosphorus is in use in some crowded offices for the same purpose; but all this is not without danger, as ozone in excess is a deadly poison, and until we have the means of determining its presence quantitatively there can be little hope of its being utilised to any great extent.

Three practical points, however, in relation to ozone are now well known :—

1. The more constant its influence in a given air and within certain limits, the greater its relative amount; the higher the degree of salubrity of the district.

2. That this is accounted for by its power of destroying hurtful gases.

3. When only present in *small quantities*, it promotes the growth of microbes.

Some of the more important physical conditions of the atmosphere have now been briefly alluded to, and this brings us to the consideration of their influence upon the living body.

A great field of inquiry of the most interesting and instructive nature here opens before us, and one which will be found to yield the highest practical results in the application of climatic conditions to the cure of disease. In following up this inquiry, it is not, however, with the hope of our being able to find any one climate which exerts such a special influence upon disease, as will give a particular district complete immunity from any known disease, or class of diseases; but that by a careful observation of the *sum* of climatic influences upon the inhabitants of any country or district we may discover a fair means of judging what morbid processes produced by one climate are likely to be hindered by another. Climatology then, to be of any practical value to medicine, must be taken in its widest sense, and must embrace the consideration of climate and soil together; and in order that the true results of the influence of these upon health and disease may be ascertained other probable factors have also to be examined, so that the effects of defective drainage, bad water, and other unsanitary conditions may not be put down to climate, which we cannot alter to any considerable degree, but traced to their true sources, which in many cases are capable of being remedied.

The question regarding the influence of geological formation and the chemical and mineralogical character of the soil upon prevailing diseases has been very keenly and very ably discussed in the cases of goitre and cretinism, but without any conclusion being arrived at of a satisfactory nature. Many distinguished observers have long held that the prevalence of these diseases was not due to mere limestone rock, but to the presence exclusively of magnesia in it; while others are equally convinced that their occurrence endemically depends upon metal-yielding rocks, and that the reason why they prevail in districts where the soil contains an abundance of magnesia is that that rock is frequently rich in sulphuret of iron; and attention has also been called to the fact that in some soils where malaria prevails iron is found in considerable quantity. As regards phthisis the clearest proof has been obtained that the disease prevails upon clayey, impermeable soils to a much greater extent than upon granite, limestone, or gravel, although in some instances the argument appears to tell the other way. So far, then, no decided conclusion has been arrived at from an examination of the geological formation of a district, or the chemical and mineralogical character of its soil.

Two important facts, however, have been ascertained in relation to goitre and malaria.

1. The influence of locality as a cause of these diseases; and

2. The influence of drainage and consequent drying of the soil in diminishing their frequency and intensity.

Referring to the first of these—the influence of locality, as a cause—Hirsch, in his classical work speaking of goitre says, " Incontrovertible proof of the influence of locality upon the production of goitre is furnished by the fact that healthy persons coming into goitrous spots from non-goitrous places not unfrequently contract the disease after a longer or shorter stay, and sometimes after a very short stay ; secondly, by the fact that a change of locality has been found to be the most certain means of overcoming the disease, or preventing its further development; and thirdly, that in regions where goitre is endemic, the animals also are affected by it, especially the domestic animals, such as dogs, cats, goats, sheep, pigs, horses, and mules." Regarding malaria the same experience is continually met with throughout Italy, notably on the Roman Campagna, in the Tuscan Maremma, and other well-known centres of malarial infection. Italians coming from their healthy homes in the mountains to tend their flocks or reap the crops on the Campagna around Rome succumb to malaria in great numbers—the death-rate among them in bad seasons running up as high as 10 per cent. In the Maremma, and especially in the districts of Orbetello and Grosetto, the inhabitants of some of the towns on the plains have to seek refuge in the mountains for several months every year, although during a recent visit which I paid to the Maremma I could in no instance discover that the lower animals were affected by the poison. At the Manganese mines on Monte Argentario in the immediate vicinity of Orbetello, where a large number of English horses are employed in the works, no case of malarious fever has occurred in the stables, although many of the men attending to them have suffered severely. These stables are now completely surrounded by belts of thriving Eucalyptus trees, and for some time the health of the horse keepers has shown a very decided improvement, with a marked diminution both in the frequency and intensity of the cases of malarious fever.

The second fact relating to the decrease of these diseases following the drainage of the soil is one of the highest practical importance, and applies not only to goitre and malaria, but also to phthisis, and, indeed, to the general well-being and health of every community, outbreaks of typhoid fever and diphtheria having been found to have a close relation to the height of the subsoil water and consequent dampness of soil. Where the moisture of the soil is great, and liable to considerable fluctuation, a very marked influence upon the prevailing diseases and upon the death-rate of a district has been observed. Wet soil, therefore, is anything but a matter of indifference to the well-being of the residents upon it, and a marked change for the better has been the invariable experience when the subsoil has been dried by drainage or in some other manner.

In England and throughout the whole of Europe there is the most abundant evidence that the public health has improved when the evil of ground water has been overcome, and the decrease of goitre, phthisis, and malaria, in districts where for centuries they had prevailed indigenously, have been justly associated with the improvements carried out in the drying of the subsoil.

CHAPTER II.

Configuration of the Coast of Italy—The Mediterranean—The City of Rome—The Campagna—Rome as a Winter Residence—Annual Mean Temperature—Rainfall—Prevailing Winds—Ozone—Prevailing Diseases in England and Italy—Malarial Cases in Male and Female Hospitals in Rome—Diphtheria and Croup—Proportion of Acute to Chronic Diseases in Italy—Degenerative Changes.

ONE of the most important factors in the climate of Italy, as well as one of the most remarkable external features of the country, consists in the peculiar configuration of the land and its relations to the Mediterranean. From Venice, on the east coast, to Ventimiglia, on the west, the coast-line measures nearly 3,000 miles in its innumerable windings upon itself, forming those countless baylets and bays, amongst them Lerici, the home of Shelley, and Naples, the greatest and grandest of them all, which are the delight and wonder of travellers. While from Bardonecchia, in the north, to Reggio, in the south, vast mountain-chains, like gigantic vertebræ, run down its centre. Thus all but entirely surrounded by the Mediterranean—a great inland sea with narrow inlets to the Atlantic and the Black Sea, and through the Suez Canal into the Red Sea—its climate presents features almost peculiar to itself, while the deep blue horizon tells of the saltness of its encircling ocean, at once the indication and the cause of much of the beauty of Italian skies and the purity of Italian air. The great influence of the Mediterranean upon the climate of Italy is due to two main causes—

1. The extreme saltness of its waters, and
2. Their high and equable temperature.

The waters of the Mediterranean are the saltest of all great seas, and this is due to the fact that the supply of fresh water received by it is much less than can supply the immense volume of water lost by evaporation. The influence of the sun is so great that in the course of years the Mediterranean, owing to its loss of water, would be a sea of salt were it not for the fact that a vast stream of Atlantic water, fed by the polar glaciers, is constantly flowing into the Straits of Gibraltar. The effect of this high degree of saltness is to cause the waters of the Mediterranean to absorb with great avidity moisture from the air, and to hold it with great tenacity, thus rendering the atmosphere around it both clear and dry. But another point of equal importance to climatologists is the equability of its temperature. During the winter months the temperature of the Mediterranean, at a depth of less than 30 feet, varies from 50 to 60 degrees Fahr., and the air above it is correspondingly warm, so that the air is warm as well as dry, and there being few hot and cold streams existing and meeting in the atmosphere, there is less vapour thrown down in the form of rain. It is easy, therefore, to see how the climate of Italy is tempered by this great body of warm water surrounding it nearly on all sides; and though the influence is felt more particularly along the coasts, yet, from the remarkable configuration of the country already referred to, the climate of the whole of Italy is more or less affected by it, and the results are seen in the type of diseases which more especially prevail throughout the kingdom, and which are nowhere more marked than in the capital itself. While, however, there is this powerful influence constantly at work over the whole length and breadth of Italy, producing its remarkable effects upon disease and presenting results of the deepest practical importance in relation to the therapeutics of climate, there are other agencies of a more local nature which affect the health of a particular city or district. Of Rome this may be said to be pre-eminently true, as there are conditions existing peculiar to itself which do not occur in or around any other great city in Europe.

The geographical position of the city of Rome, at the Observatory of the Roman College, so long adorned by the accomplished and renowned Padre Secchi, is lat. 41° 53′ 52″ N., long. 12° 28′ 40″ E. of Greenwich, and though still called the City of the Seven Hills, the same relations do not exist now between the city and the seven hills as existed in the days of the kings, during the Republic, or under the Empire. In the earliest of these periods the centre of life and activity was the Palatine, which immediately overlooked the Forum, and in later times the common people were gradually driven from it to make room for the wealthier citizens who, drawn hither by accounts of its purer air and greater healthiness, began to erect those villas which afterwards became so famous. It was here that Cicero excited so much envy by the grandeur of his house, and it was to the slopes of the Palatine that Augustus ventured to remove the royal residence from the Forum below.

From this time it became the abode of the Cæsars, and the royal palace grew in extent and magnificence under each succeeding emperor, until nearly the whole of the hill was occupied by it, the ruins of which are now one of the chief attractions of the Italian capital.

The seven hills surround the city in the form of an irregular crescent, although it may be said to occupy only four of them, while the remaining three are left in ruins or covered by gardens.

The Tiber divides the city into two unequal parts. Entering the line of the walls close to the north gate, it winds half round the city, and after a swift course of more than 20 miles, pours itself into the Tyrrhenian Sea. The mean elevation of Rome above the sea is about 90 feet. Some of the hills are considerably higher, the Esquiline being nearly 190 feet, while the Janiculum, on the Vatican side of the river, rises to a height of more than 300 feet. The most important feature, however, in the topography of Rome, and one which influences its climate and health more than any other, is the Campagna, which may be said to surround it. Situated nearly in the centre of this magnificent, extensive, but dreaded territory, it is supposed to be encircled with a most deadly atmosphere, and the mere name of the Campagna is calculated to awaken the most disquieting feelings in the minds of those who have been warned against exposing themselves to its poisonous vapours.

To the residents all this excites the most genuine surprise, as to them a drive on the Campagna is one of the most delightful, while it is one of the most healthful that can be taken in Rome. Why then all this fear on the part of the stranger? Is there any foundation for the warnings which he has received? or is it merely a fancy which will not bear investigation, or what is more likely still, is it due to those who have a purpose to serve in the solicitude they manifest for the safety of the visitor who is bold enough to venture into a city where, as Hawthorne says, "fever walks arm-in-arm with us, and where death awaits us at the end of our walk;" or as expressed by another, "a city which is surrounded by the *dismal swamp* of the Campagna?" If what these and other writers who have used equally strong language in depicting the climate of Rome be true, then there is more than reason for the alarm felt by strangers who have yielded to the fascination which Rome has always exercised for the cultured mind, and there is ample ground for the solicitude shown for their safety by their relatives and friends. These are important matters and require clear and thorough investigation, and in the chapters upon "The Unhealthiness of Rome," and "How to live in Rome," I will endeavour to show as fully, and in as strict accordance with the facts as I can, where the truth appears to lie.

This is not the first time that the attempt has been made to remove misapprehensions which prevail regarding the climate of Rome, or to point out dangers which have to be avoided, more especially by unacclimatized visitors, who for a time take up their abode within its walls. For a period of more than twelve years I had the opportunity of observing in Florence some of the effects of a winter's residence in Rome upon persons who had visited Italy for the first time, and were therefore unacclimatized. During the same period, a considerable number of cases of so-called Roman fever came under my care. The experience of these twelve years, compared with experience gained during the past three years, since my practice was transferred to Rome, has led me to believe that drinking water is one of the probable modes by which malaria may enter the system. I will give the reasons for this belief when speaking of Malaria and the Water Supply of Rome.

The meteorological features of the climate of Rome have led to its being classed amongst temperate, moist, inland climates, having indeed a *quasi* maritime character. Sometimes it has been described as a dry climate possessing the softness of a warm and moist atmosphere. So far as one can attempt to define it, the latter description is not inapt, for while the amount of absolute moisture is somewhat high, showing a mean annual average of nearly 10, the mean relative moisture rarely exceeds 66, and this latter fact, coupled with the prevailing high temperature which shows an annual mean of nearly 60° Fahr., readily accounts for a high degree of moisture existing in the air, imparting a softness and mildness to it which, however, seldom gives evidence of its presence by appearing as fogs or mists.

The Roman climate therefore is essentially a warm one. The most recent observations give the following particulars :—

The annual mean temperature 59·5° Fahr.

,, Winter ,, ,, 45·3° ,,
,, Spring ,, ,, 57·3° ,,
,, Summer ,, ,, 74·5° ,,
,, Autumn ,, ,, 61·2° ,,

The coldest month in the year is January, while the two hottest are July and August, and they are nearly equal in temperature, August being a trifle cooler than July. June and September are also nearly alike, while October marks a decided fall in the thermometer which goes on till February, when it begins to rise again.

The highest degree of heat recorded in recent years was 98·2° Fahr., and during the same period the lowest point reached by the thermometer was 21·2° Fahr. The barometric pressure has an annual mean of 29·82 inches, the mean variation between the extreme points being less than two degrees. While, however, the average temperature in winter is fairly high, the cold is frequently felt as intense, especially during the tramontana.

The next important element in the climatology of Rome is the humidity of the atmosphere. The comparatively high mean temperature just referred to, together with the Tiber, and other evaporating surfaces, and the prevalence of the south-east wind in winter, and the south-west in summer, suggest the presence of a considerable amount of absolute moisture in the air, which, as we have already seen, has an annual average of 10°. The average amount of rainfall, and number of rainy days, are given below.

	Amount of Rain in m.m.	Number of Rainy Days.
December	81·85	11·5
January	74·16	11·8
February	59·65	10·5
March	64·44	11·5
April	60·39	10·6
May	54·76	0·7
June	38·03	7·5
July	16·73	3·6
August	28·57	5·0
September	69·97	8·6
October	105·96	11·2
November	114·35	12·8

The above table shows that the annual rainfall is about 29 inches, and is distributed over 114 days, although nearly one half of the whole amount falls during the autumn months. The table further shows that there is in Rome a tolerably well marked dry and wet season. The former extending from May till September, and the latter from October till April. The mean relative humidity for the year is 66·6, while in summer it is as low as 39, and during the winter it is not unusual to see a difference of 4 or 5 degrees between the wet and dry bulbs, and of course in summer much greater.

Two years ago I attended a young gentleman in the Hotel Quirinal, who was a victim to asthma complicated with rheumatism. Damp weather invariably brought on an attack of asthma, but not so the rheumatic symptoms, which only seemed to increase when dampness came on suddenly after dry weather. So constantly was he reminded of his infirmities by the alternation of wet and dry weather that he became an expert in observing these meteorological changes. During his stay in Rome, which extended from the middle of April till the end of May, he suffered very slightly from attacks of asthma and scarcely at all from rheumatism. From a series of very careful observations which he made, it was found that the mean difference between the wet and dry bulbs in his own room was 4·9° Fahr. and the maximum 7·3° Fahr. Whenever the difference fell to about 3° Fahr. he began to experience a difficulty of breathing accompanied by wheezing, and between this point and 1·5° Fahr. the attack invariably came on. He further observed that even during and after sharp thunder showers the difference between the bulbs stood so high as to enable him to go about freely and to make the remark that "a shower of rain in Rome appeared to affect him less than elsewhere."

The following is a table of the prevailing winds with their relative frequency in a thousand times :—

	North or Tramontana.	North East or Greco.	East or Levante.	South East or Scirocco.	South or Mezzogiorno.	South West or Libeccio.	West or Ponente.	North West or Maestro.
Winter	564	45	68	27	188	31	63	14
Spring	291	22	44	19	303	90	206	25
Summer	239	19	20	7	245	151	291	28
Autumn	388	32	68	23	249	72	143	25
Whole Year	370	30	50	19	246	86	176	23

The north wind is the predominating wind in winter and autumn, the south in spring and the west in summer. While the north wind prevails, the weather is generally cold and dry, and it usually indicates fine settled weather. When it follows a continued rainless scirocco, it may, however, bring rain, and is then called Tramontana *torbida*, or *sporca*. This *wet* north wind never lasts for more than a day or two. The South wind is moist and warm, while the West, which prevails in the sultry summer months, comes with delightful freshness from the sea. It is usually a dry wind, although sometimes rainy weather accompanies it, and when this happens, a warm south wind is sure to have prevailed before it. The south-west wind in summer is a wet wind, and the south-east or scirocco in winter is nearly always wet. Italians generally call *all* south winds Scirocco, and hence this wind, so *unliked* by the strong and healthy, is said to prevail frequently, whereas a glance at the foregoing table will show that it is the least frequent of all the winds in Rome.

The amount of ozone in the air of Rome is very considerable, but not in sufficient quantity to cause irritation of the mucous surfaces of the chest, as is evidenced by the fact that chronic bronchitis, affections of the lungs themselves, and even phthisis in its very early stages usually do well there. The proportion of ozone, as might be expected, is greater during the spring and summer months than it is in the winter. Throughout the year 1877—the year for which I have the fullest data—there was no day when ozone was absent from the air. Sometimes there would be as much as 8·5 and never less than 1·2. In the spring and summer the mean amount is about 5·2, while in autumn and winter, it is not more than 4·0. As has been mentioned already, we know very little about the precise physiological effects of this curious and interesting agent. The most general opinion as to its production is that its chief natural sources are sunlight and vegetation, the former probably determining its amount in sea air, and the latter that in forest air, or in districts covered with healthy vegetation. The influence of wind is also important, as ozone is less in stagnant air than when wind prevails, and moreover, it is well known that epidemics are apt to spread more rapidly when the atmosphere is calm, than when in motion. It is not unusual to find that test papers, exposed close to buildings having a windward position, are not affected, while if placed in the line of the wind they will speedily be acted upon. According to Grellois it is more abundant over a marsh than elsewhere, and from experiments made with the organic matter, in the air over marshes it was found that ozone did not destroy the organic matter, while the organic matter was thought to destroy quinine.

On the other hand, Uhle says that malaria accumulates in the air at night from the non-production of ozone by the sun's rays. While, therefore, there is some difference of opinion among observers regarding the production of ozone and its effects upon marsh air, there is considerable unanimity, as stated in a previous page, regarding its influence in purifying the air, in the degree of salubrity of a place corresponding with the amount of ozone in its air, as well as that the amount of ozone in the air inhaled corresponds with the supposed most important function of the blood corpuscles (Braun).

There can be little doubt, that to it in some measure is due the favourable position in the matter of healthiness which Rome occupies, when compared with other great European cities. Its position, indeed, in this respect, is all the more favourable when we take into consideration the numerous factors which have been at work for centuries tending to increase its unhealthiness, and especially the utter neglect until recently of all sanitary matters, together with its subtropical climate. Having to contend against such powerful influences, the wonder is that Rome compares so well with other continental cities, and when the scheme for improving the Campagna, which has now become law, is fully in operation, and the sanitary improvements which are now being vigorously carried out are finished, there is every hope that the sanitary position of Rome among great cities will be higher still.

The chief elements in the climate of Rome may therefore be summed up as follows :—

The comparatively high mean *annual* and *winter* temperature, and the abundance of sunshine, the temperature being subject to great and sudden changes in winter and spring. The high amount of absolute moisture, and the comparatively low degree of relative moisture, together with the presence of a large number of evaporating surfaces and the south-east wind in winter, with the south-west in summer, —both moisture-laden winds.

The prevalence of the undermentioned principal winds in the following order.

    a. North or Tramontana, cold and usually dry.
    b. South or Mezzogiorno, warm and moist.
    c. West or Ponente, occasionally moist.
    d. South-west or Libeccio, warm and moist.
    e. East or Levante, dry.
    f. North-east, or Greco, cool and dry.
    g. North-west or Maestro (Mistral), dry.
    h. South-east or Scirroco, warm and moist.

The abundance of ozone, and the situation of the city in the centre of the vast undulating Campagna which is formed of volcanic strata, having a peculiarly porous superficial surface which is covered, where uncultivated, during spring and early summer, with a crop of natural hay. A thoughtful consideration of these main features in the climate of Rome will readily suggest reasons why the city should be one of more than average healthiness. For the present I do not take into consideration the flaws in its sanitary condition nor its abundant supply of wholesome water, as these are treated of in chapters further on, but simply the meteorological features of its climate. The high amount and degree of sunlight intensifying all the chemical actions in the animal body, the constant presence in the air of a considerable proportion of ozone acting upon and destroying deleterious gases, and a certain quantity of moisture in its warm atmosphere rendering it soothing, and thus highly beneficial in chronic bronchitis and in various other chest and throat affections.

Our next inquiry is how this climate affects the health of the inhabitants as seen in the types of disease which ordinarily prevail among them. In a paper which appeared in the *Practitioner*, many years ago, I pointed out what seemed a remarkable difference between the types of disease prevailing in Florence, and, indeed, throughout the kingdom of Italy, and those usually prevalent in England and northern climes generally. In Florence I found that the great bulk of medical practice was made up of acute diseases, whereas, in England, the reverse was true, and chronic diseases were much more common than acute. Not only is this the case, but acute diseases in England usually run a much slower course than they do in Italy. There is, in Italy, a striking increase in the intensity of all vital processes, and this increased intensity is not more shown in the rapidity with which acute diseases, such as pneumonia, run their course, than by the speedy benefit derived in more chronic cases in which the processes of tissue change require hastening. What is true of Italy in this respect is particularly true of Rome, as I will now endeavour to show. It is impossible to compare the prevailing diseases of Rome with those of any of our large home cities; or even to compare in as accurate a manner as could be wished the mortality of so important an index of the health of a given population as the class of zymotic diseases presents, because the nomenclature and classification of diseases are not the same in the two countries, and of course the calculations cannot be made for the same causes of death. I have thought, therefore, that by giving a few specimens of well-marked disease as examples, a truer idea of the effects of the climate of Rome upon health and disease would be ascertained than if the attempt was made, under existing circumstances, to compare the whole list of diseases throughout. The most recent comparison with which I am acquainted, of death causes and prevailing diseases based upon statistical evidence in Italy and in England, is that made by the late Dr. King Chambers, and refers more especially to the cities of Genoa and Milan; and it will be interesting to observe that in the case of Rome, except in the one item of malarial fever, which is due to local causes, the prevalent diseases are, in the main, much the same as those found to prevail in North Italy, showing, as has been already observed, that there are certain climatal conditions which may be said to exert a common influence over the kingdom of Italy generally.

TABLE I.
Comparison of selected Causes of Death in Italy and England.

	LONDON.		GENOA.	
	No. of Deaths.	Proportion to total Deaths.	No. of Deaths.	Proportion to total Deaths.
Total from all causes................	67,371	—	4,303	—
Typhus, typhoid, small-pox, measles, scarlatina, whooping cough & croup	12,915	1 in 5·2	779	1 in 5·6
Chronic. Anasarca or general dropsy .... Nephria and kidney disease.... "Asthma" and "bronchitis," or chronic affections of the respiratory organs, except consumption...............	6,552	1 in 10	215	1 in 20
Pulmonary consumption	7,871	1 in 8	318	1 in 13
Epilepsy...........................	373	1 in 180	17	1 in 253
Aneurism	103	—	20	—
Chronic affections of heart	2,840	1 in 27	126	1 in 33
Cancer	1,335	1 in 50	67	1 in 64
Total of chief chronic diseases as above	20,572	1 in 3·2	761	1 in 5·6
Acute. Acute affections of digestive viscera or "enteritis," "gastritis," "diarrhœa," and "dysentery"...............	2,310	1 in 30·3	480	1 in 8·9
Acute affections of respiratory organs, or "laryngitis," "pleurisy," and "pneumonia" ...	4,021	1 in 16	450	1 in 16
Cephalitis, encephalitis, meningitis, and spinitis	566	1 in 119	72	1 in 59
Apoplexy and cerebral congestion	1,653	1 in 40	192	1 in 22
Acute inflammation of the organs of circulation, or pericarditis	111	1 in 606	97	1 in 44
Total of chief acute diseases as above not including zymotics ...	8,661	1 in 7·7	1,291	1 in 3·3

TABLE II.
Comparison of Hospital Patients.

		At Ospitale Maggiore in three years		At St. Mary's Hospital, London, in nine years.	
		Number Admitted.	Proportion to Total.	Number Admitted.	Proportion to Total.
Chronic.	All medical diseases	61,761	—	7,319	—
	Bright's disease, or general dropsy, with diseased kidneys	22	1 in 2,807	232	1 in 31
	Anasarca without diseased kidneys, dependent on diseased heart, chronic bronchitis, or no known cause	776	1 in 78	74	1 in 98
	Ascites*	625	1 in 98	54	1 in 135
	Hepatitis*	464	1 in 133	9	1 in 813
	"Chronic bronchitis," or "bronchorrhœa"	7	1 in 8,823	224	1 in 32
	Pulmonary consumption	1,551	1 in 39	527	1 in 13
	Chronic brain disease, softening, &c.	0	—	12	—
	Aneurism of aorta	4	1 in 15440	29	1 in 252
	Organic disease of heart	1,717	1 in 35	260	1 in 25
	Total of the above diseases, except hepatitis	4,702	1 in 13	1,412	1 in 5
Acute.	Enteritis, gastritis, gastro-enteritis, diarrhœa and dysentery	7,415	1 in 8	90	1 in 81
	Pneumonia and pleurisy	4,904	1 in 12	330	1 in 22
	Bronchitis (febrile)	5,668	1 in 10	245	1 in 29
	Encephalitis, meningitis	513	1 in 120	29	1 in 252
	Noteo myelitis, or inflammation of the spinal cord	475	1 in 130	1	1 in 7,319
	Apoplexy and sanguineous congestion of the brain	230	1 in 268	90	1 in 81
	Pericarditis, endocarditis	316	1 in 195	119	1 in 53
	Erysipelas	1,000	1 in 61	69	1 in 106
	Rheumatic fever, acute and subacute rheumatism	3,203	1 in 19	835	1 in 8
	Zymotic continued fever, to wit, typhus, typhoid, gastric, catarrhal, angiostenic, and typho-puerperal	8,266	1 in 7	471	1 in 15
	Total of the above acute diseases	31,950	1 in 1·9	2,293	1 in 3·1

* Hepatitis is placed here simply to have it beside ascites, and not because it is looked upon as a chronic disease.

Turning to Rome itself, an item in the death-rate appears which has not been met with in the two preceding tables, and one which forms the largest proportion of admissions into the great public hospitals. This item is malarial fever in one or other of its various forms, and while it is impossible to obtain reliable evidence of the exact number of cases actually occurring in and around the city, owing to these fevers not being included in the list for which compulsory notification exists, sufficient data will be found in some of the reports of the large medical hospitals to prove what diseases appear in largest numbers amongst their admissions, or figure highest in their statistics of mortality, and therefore may be supposed to give a tolerably accurate idea of the prevailing diseases of the population, as well as any special features which may be peculiarly characteristic of them.

A few years ago, Professor Scalzi, of Rome, prepared a most able and valuable report illustrative of the influence of weather on the production of malarial fevers and acute diseases of the respiratory organs based upon the statistics of the two great male and female medical hospitals of Rome.

From this report I take the following tables:—

Table III.

Number of admissions into the Santo Spirito Hospital (Male Medical) of malarial fevers and acute diseases of the lungs in 1877:—

Months.	Malarial Fevers.			Pleurisy, Pneumonia and Pleuro-pneumonia.	Other Diseases	Total admission.
	Intermittent.	Pernicious	Total.			
December	46	4	50	15	193	258
January	54	1	55	22	195	272
February	41	3	44	21	265	330
March	44	5	49	24	208	281
April	66	5	71	26	221	318
May	58	1	59	16	197	272
June	57	2	59	12	198	269
July	169	1	170	7	214	391
August	300	10	310	0	212	522
September	301	5	306	5	217	528
October	226	1	227	16	175	418
November	97	0	97	10	215	322
Total	12,261	275	12,536	970	3,947	17,453

N.B.—Out of a total number of 17,453 cases admitted into the Male Medical Hospital, no less than 13,506 were due to malarial fevers and acute diseases of the chest alone, making in round numbers more than three-fourths of the total admissions for the year, and if we add to these figures the numbers of the *acute* disorders, for which, however, I have not sufficiently clear and reliable statistics, such diseases, for example, as enteritis, diarrhœa, meningitis, and acute affections of the heart, the total number of acute diseases cannot be much under four-fifths of the whole admissions for the year.

TABLE IV.

Number of admissions into the San Giovanni Hospital (Female Medical) of malarial fevers and acute diseases of the lungs in 1877:—

Months.	Malarial Fevers.			Pleurisy, Pneumonia and Pleuro-pneumonia.	Other Diseases	Total Admissions.
	Intermittent.	Pernicious	Total			
December	46	4	50	15	193	258
January	54	1	55	22	195	272
February	41	3	44	21	265	330
March	44	5	49	24	208	281
April	66	5	71	26	221	318
May	58	1	59	16	197	272
June	57	2	59	12	198	269
July	169	1	170	7	214	391
August	300	10	310	0	212	522
September	301	5	306	5	217	528
October	226	1	227	16	175	418
November	97	0	97	10	215	322
Total	1,459	38	1,497	174	2,510	4,181

N.B.—Out of a total number of 4,181 cases of all kinds admitted into the Female Hospital, 1,671 were due to malarial fever and acute affections of the lungs. The proportion of acute disease to chronic in this Table is not so great, as was found to exist in the Male Medical Hospital. The difference, however is found in the number of fever cases and not among the affections of the lungs, the latter being almost equal in proportion to those among the men. The reason why so much less fever prevails among the women is that few of them are agricultural labourers, and are therefore much less exposed to malarial influences than the male population. If, however, we add the numbers of acute cases of other diseases, the proportion of acute to chronic disease will still remain relatively high.

The element in the two preceding tables which is subject to the greatest variation is the malarial. Some seasons are notoriously unhealthy, and the number of fever cases is greatly increased. Thus, in 1864, out of 11,679 persons admitted into the Santo Spirito Hospital, 5,809 were affected with malaria, or about one-half of the entire number. In 1865 the fever cases amounted to rather more than a third of the whole, and in 1877 to three-fourths of the total number of patients for the year. Severe winters, too, naturally increase the number of lung affections. As, for instance, the winter 1879-80, which was an unusually cold one, proved very fatal to a large number of persons suffering from affections of the chest. From December, 1879, till March, 1880, no fewer than 1,718 having succumbed to inflammation of the lungs and bronchitis in the short period between those dates. Following ague and diseases of the lungs, the next important affection in the order of frequency is diphtheria, which shows a rather high mortality. In the five years prior to 1880 there were 1,476 deaths registered as due to this cause alone, but as no distinction is made between diphtheria and the various affections frequently classed under the name croup, it is impossible to say how many of these cases were due to true diphtheria.

Indeed, it is not unlikely that several affections of the throat and windpipe are included at the registration office under the one term. From a considerable experience, I am inclined to believe that so-called membranous croup is diphtheria, and were this the only disease mixed up with the latter, the statistics would not be materially influenced one way or the other.

Enteritis, dysentery, diarrhœa, rheumatism, and consumption all occupy important places among the causes of death; while, however, measles, scarlatina, and whooping cough, generally speaking, run a very mild course. My present object being to endeavour to show the relation which the climate of Rome bears to its prevalent diseases, I have only chosen those which are more especially apt to be affected by weather or some local element in the climate, and included measles and scarlatina, as well as whooping cough, which, though having specific sources, seem to be so influenced by the Roman climate as to present features differing considerably from those seen in other Continental cities, more especially in the less dangerous forms, which they almost invariably assume. From what has been stated, it will be seen that acute diseases prevail throughout Italy, and particularly in Rome, in a greater degree than they do in England, and, I believe, in northern climates generally; and not only so, but chronic diseases, which form so large a proportion of medical practice in England and other countries, are comparatively rare in Italy. This contrast is the more striking, the more decidedly chronic and degenerative the disease is. It is not easy to present these facts in a tabular form, the statistics are very numerous regarding certain points in the inquiry, while they are meagre as regards others; moreover, it is impossible to know exactly the number of cases of any given disease except it be of those only who apply for relief at the various hospitals, or come under the scope of compulsory notification; and besides, it may not infrequently happen that the subject of an old standing disease is cut off by an acute attack, or an acute disease registered as such might slowly pass into a chronic form. These are difficulties which, as matters now exist, are not easily overcome, and render even a proximate accuracy impossible. Yet no one can study the very few and imperfect statistics which I have given without being struck with the fact of the great prevalence, in Italy, of acute diseases, and the equally remarkable fact of the absence of so many chronic diseases due to degenerative changes, which are so numerous in all our homelands. This is a fruitful field for inquiry, and Italy, from several peculiar and decided features in its climate, affords scope for the investigation of the effects of climate upon certain types of disease in a greater degree than any other country with which I am acquainted.

. Every practitioner of any standing in Italy will bear testimony to the truth of what has been stated, and those of my brethren practising in Rome will readily admit the rarity of the occurrence of such diseases as Bright's disease, diabetes, hepatic disease, and those due to alcoholic excesses, which number so many victims during the course of a single year in England. It would seem therefore that acute diseases in Rome are not so apt to pass into a chronic or degenerative stage as they are in England, and that chronic ailments in themselves occur so seldom, or give so little trouble, that they rarely come under the care of a physician; and this fact holds true of all classes, of the poor as well as the rich, so that the influence which brings about this result is not confined to any one portion of the population, but is felt by all, and therefore in all probability is due to climate and not to any social rank. If further inquiry establish the truth of this statement, if those chronic diseases which are so fatal in England are proved to be in reality the reverse in Italy, may it not be a climate suitable for their cure? and if suitable to the cure of these diseases, is there not the hope that by a timely *change of air* many of those cases hitherto looked upon as hopeless may be found to yield to such a climate as Rome affords?

CHAPTER III.

The Unhealthiness of Rome—Typhoid in Rome and Paris—A Death in Dresden—Sanitary Condition of Rome—Roman Churches and their Burying Grounds—Pernicious Influence of Stagnant Pools—Modern Closets—*A Sanitary Festa*—Malarial Fever—Unhealthy Dwellings—The Jews in the Ghetto—*Febbre Perniciosa*—Diphtheria and Small-pox—Deaths from Typhoid in Italy and London—Number of English and American Visitors in Rome—Roman Wells.

Two hundred years ago Dr. Gideon Harvey, writing of Rome, says: "The air at Rome is likewise very pernicious, especially all the summer, at which time, as I was informed, no person will hazard to travel towards Naples for fear of incurring that dangerous fever which the change of air brings unavoidably on them, especially among those who return from Naples to Rome, among whom scarce one in a hundred escapes." From Dr. Harvey's day down to our own the most earnest attempts have been made to vilify the sanitary reputation of Rome. Especially has this been the case in recent years, and writers of all nationalities, but particularly English and American, have vied with each other in their efforts to find language sufficiently strong to show their dislike of Rome and its detestable and deadly climate. Perhaps no city in Europe has been so abused in this respect as Rome has, or afforded a more favourite theme upon which authors have delighted to dwell. The result of all this has been a most natural one; Rome is dreaded by everybody, and it is enough for any one to have passed through it, for the city to be credited with almost any disease with which he may happen to be affected for some time afterwards, however far away he may be before such disease might show itself. Thus it not infrequently appears in the obituary column of the *Times* or other well-known journal that such a person died of fever *caught at Rome.* As fever prevails there as in other great cities, the possibility of visitors being affected by it is as true of Rome as it is of other places, but why it should be supposed to be only true of Rome and not of other cities as well, is more difficult to imagine. In the case of travellers who may have visited many cities in Italy—Rome among the number — and continued their tour through Germany and France, how could it be said of any of them who might afterwards be stricken with typhoid fever that it was *caught at Rome?* as if no other city which they may have visited was capable of producing such a result; and yet it is just in cases of this kind that I have been able to trace such an inference as the above to, and is all the more to be regretted, because if the truth were told, Rome would probably be found to have a lower death-rate from typhoid fever than any of the continental capitals, and this remark is especially true, when the number of deaths from typhoid in Rome and Paris are compared.*

The following case is not without interest as showing to what lengths such a method of reasoning may sometimes carry one. Four years ago I had under my care in Florence a young lady who had been visiting Southern Italy. She had spent a fortnight in Naples, and towards the end of her stay was suddenly attacked with diarrhœa; as soon as she was supposed to be able to travel she came on to

---

* During the year 1882 typhoid fever caused in Paris 3,276 deaths, out of a total number of 58,674. In 1881 the deaths were 2,120, out of a total of 56,820. Thus the mortality from typhoid fever was greater by 1 per 1,000 in 1882 than in the preceding year. Moreover, during the past ten years, the total number of deaths has presented a progressive increase. Ten years ago the mortality oscillated between 21 and 23 per 1,000, in 1881 it was 25·37 per 1,000, and in 1882 it was 26·55 per 1,000. Of these 3,276 deaths due to typhoid fever, 1,449 occurred in the hospitals and 1,827 at the home of patients.

Rome. The malady returned on the journey, and she arrived worse than when she left Naples. She remained in Rome only for a couple of days, during which time she felt comparatively well; but such was her dread of being ill there that her physician thought it prudent to send her to Florence. When I saw her she was suffering from severe gastric derangement. There was tenderness over the liver with slight fulness, and the spleen was decidedly enlarged; but the temperature was normal. In the course of a few days she appeared very much in her usual health. After remaining in Florence for about a week she left for Germany, travelling over the Brenner *viâ* Innsbrück. I heard nothing more of her until I received a newspaper notice of her death, which occurred in Dresden two months after she left Florence, the cause of death being stated to be due to *fever caught at Rome*. Such a narrative as this requires no comment. Unhappily, however, it is far from being an uncommon one, and a general though vague belief all but universally prevails regarding the dangers to which travellers are exposed when, so far braving all the statements by which they have been sought to be convinced, they yield to the fascination which the name of the city of the Seven Hills has always exercised from its earliest days. However, while thousands of visitors every year are thus found who apparently throw aside their fears, yet it is a fact that there is no city in Europe which they enter with so many disquieting feelings and so much trembling as they do when they come within the walls of the Italian capital, and these in themselves become a source of peril to visitors by rendering them more susceptible to the dangers which to some extent they already dread. Nor is it only the reports of the unhealthy condition of Rome with which they set out on their travels that visitors have to endeavour to forget, for the nearer they approach Italy the less vague do the reports become, and indeed nowhere is the unhealthiness of Rome more persistently urged upon the attention of strangers than at Genoa and Pisa, Venice and Florence. During my residence in the latter city it was amusing to observe the ways by which some of the hotel keepers endeavoured to put Rome in an unfavourable light, and the most *recent statistics* were presented in person or through the courier to show, not only how disinterested they were in the solicitude they manifested, but to prove the reliability of their facts; and it will not be surprising to learn that in a large number of instances the *statistics* carried the day, and many who had looked forward to seeing a long-cherished hope realized by a visit to the city of the Cæsars were dissuaded from such an unwise attempt, and remained in their comfortable quarters on the Arno, or sought a safer retreat than Rome elsewhere.

It is difficult to believe that all these impressions regarding the sanitary condition of Rome are without foundation; that the so-called recent statistics, which are so readily forthcoming when occasion requires are myths, produced in the interests of self, or that all the abuse to which the city has been subjected is unmerited. There surely must be a deeper reason than any of these lying at the root of this wide-spread belief, entertained by so many who have no personal interests to serve, and who cannot be said to be totally ignorant of Italy and its climate, or unfriendly to it as a nation which is rapidly making itself felt as one of the great European Powers. My own conviction is that there is some ground for it, and into the nature and extent of that ground I now propose to inquire.

This inquiry naturally divides itself into something like the following elements :—

> The present sanitary condition of Rome.
> The reason why malarial fevers and acute diseases of the lungs figure so largely in the death-rate.

The mortality from typhoid fever.

How malarial and typhoid fevers respectively affect strangers resident in the city, and

How does it happen that such a deeply rooted belief in the unhealthiness of Rome is on the increase, notwithstanding its improved sanitary condition and its gradually diminishing death-rate?

Much has been written in recent years to prove the salubrity of Rome in ancient times, and historic evidence is not awanting to show that the early Romans were thoroughly conversant with hygienic laws. The remarkable system of archaic subsoil drainage found in connection with the Roman hills, the so-called "cunicular drains" of the Campagna, the magnificent water supply of the city, which, as early as a hundred years before the Christian era was capable of supplying more than 300 million gallons daily, or about 900 gallons per head of a population the average of the present one, together prove that the Roman engineers were fully alive to the importance of those great sanitary questions which exert such a powerful influence upon the health and prosperity of a people.

While, however, the health of their city was maintained, that of the Campagna surrounding it gradually suffered from the fatal policy pursued by the Romans of carrying the inhabitants of conquered cities in the neighbourhood to Rome as slaves. Their lands were consigned to colonists, under whom they fell into a state of complete decay, the drainage was neglected, imperfect cultivation of the soil naturally followed, the Campagna relapsed into desert, and malaria began to spread over it like a deadly mantle. In time, too, vicissitudes beset the city itself. From the terrible fire during the reign of Nero, till the year 476, when the Roman Empire was broken up, the city was devastated and plundered again and again. In 600 the Bishop of Rome became Pope, and from that time onwards till the reign of Pius the Ninth, the process of gradual decay within the walls seems to have been slowly going on. The health of Rome at this period must have been far from satisfactory, but nothing certain is known, for though the Vatican published returns from one Easter to another, based upon very insufficient data and an imperfect census taken in 1853, they are completely valueless for statistical purposes.

One of the most fruitful sources of disease within the city walls during the reign of the later Popes must have been the great number of intramural burying-places. As there are no less than about 370 churches in Rome, and as each church has a separate cemetery, some idea may be formed of the extent of this danger—a danger not lessened by the fact that innumerable wells were used for the purpose of supplying water for domestic use.

To Napoleon the First, I believe, is due the credit of establishing a burying-ground outside the walls; a step which the papal authorities saw the advantage of, for gradually interments within the city were prohibited, and now no such thing is known. Another feature of equal import accomplished recently has been the closing, by an order of the municipality, of all wells within the city. In the majority of the old Roman houses these wells existed and were sunk to a considerable depth, and of course were easily polluted by the infiltration of subsoil water, while their sides, which were green with damp, became during the hot summer months a source of mischief by the unwholesome exhalations which emanated from them. The same may be said of the now ruined fountains within the grounds of many private villas. In early days their owners were possessed of vast wealth, and these fountains were miniature gushing streams; but as the general decay crept on they fell into ruin and became little more than pools of stagnant water covered by putrifying vegetation. The pernicious influence of stagnant pools of this nature in the vicinity of dwelling-houses was proved beyond doubt in an investigation which I made in Florence in 1876, when diphtheria visited the city. The first case which I saw occurred in the middle of April, and between that date and the end of May I attended in all twenty-one cases, which though generally of a mild character, proved fatal in several instances. The weather was very warm and water was not abundant. In more than two-thirds of the above number, the children who became affected spent the greater part of the day under the shade of trees in the gardens surrounding the houses in which they lived, and in *all* of these gardens there were ornamental fountains which, during the period under consideration, contained stagnant water full of decaying vegetable matter which was evidently the cause of the outbreak. No other source could be discovered, and that it was not due—in at least one of the families—to contaminated drinking-water was placed beyond doubt by the fact that the water used in the nursery was brought three times a week from Vallambrosa, one of the purest and most delightful drinking-waters in Tuscany. In Rome large numbers of these fountains are rapidly disappearing before the improvements which are everywhere throughout the city being carried out.

Another source of trouble arose from the system of drainage adopted within the houses, which was usually of the most primitive character. In some of the houses, it is true, the common privy was situated on a balcony outside the house, and however primitive in construction, it was less likely to be a source of danger from its position outside the dwelling; but in other cases it was placed not only inside the house, but actually in the kitchen itself! Frequently the small lanes and side streets were made to supplement these *conveniences*, and it is not yet so long ago since several of the main thoroughfares in the immediate neighbourhood of the Piazza di Spagna were rendered almost unfit for ladies to pass from the accumulated filth in the bye-streets which intersected them, and the *dust heaps* at their corners over which was inscribed the somewhat uneuphonious name of *Immondezzia*. These very lanes and bye-streets are now well paved and clean, and are inhabited by well-to-do citizens, as well as by many visitors—both English and American. Other dangers, too, existed in the manner by which these closets discharged themselves into the sewers or cesspools.

Many of these sewers and cesspools were built centuries ago, and their very existence forgotten; while others, which from long accumulating refuse had become entirely occluded were allowed to remain in connection with those still in use. All this is now being dealt with by the municipality and the Government in a most thorough manner. New drains of good construction are being laid where necessary throughout the city, old ones are being repaired or renewed, and the whole system of drainage is to converge to a great main sewer—so long the desideratum of Rome—along the new Tiber embankment, which will carry the sewage beyond the city before it finds its way into the river. Some danger has also arisen from many of the old privies having been converted into modern closets. An imperfect modern closet, without sufficient water, and the discharge pipes having no direct communication with the open air, is a greater danger, as is well known, than the old primitive plan, and to this cause I was able to trace two cases of typhoid during last winter. The occupants of the house, though conscious of a sickly odour in the closet and bedroom adjoining, were perfectly sure that no trouble could come from *their* closet, "*which was an English one, and of the most approved construction.*"

It can scarcely be wondered at that with such a condition of things as existed prior to 1870, Rome should have had a well-earned reputation for its unhealthiness, even although before it became the capital of the kingdom of Italy, the Papal Government had taken some steps to render it less notorious for its unsanitary condition. Some of these measures were, however, of less than doubtful utility, and tended rather to increase than diminish the unenviable reputation which it had. One of these communicated to me by my friend Mr. Shakspere Wood, the accomplished correspondent of the *Times*, is of a somewhat amusing character, and shows how the Romans of to-day are not one whit behind their ancestors in contriving to find *divertimento* in the least entertaining of subjects and on the most unlikely occasions.

"Up to a very recent period it was the custom to flood the immense Piazza Navona—then a vegetable market—with water every Sunday during the month of August. It was made a kind of popular festa. Those who kept, or could afford to hire carriages, used to drive backwards and forwards through the water, stirring up the refuse of decayed vegetables below, while the poorer sat around in crowds enjoying the fun. After the sluices were opened, some of the accumulated refuse of the week was carried off. The remainder, soaked with water, lay and rotted in the sweltering August sun, and yet people wondered why August should be so unhealthy a month, or so many people be struck down with fever."

Rome having superior attractions to any of the other Italian cities, naturally drew within its walls a larger number of foreigners. This exciting the jealousy of neighbouring cities, they lost no opportunity of making known whatever might prove detrimental to its sanitary reputation and thus, if possible, cause a diminution in the number of strangers visiting it. The exaggerated reports circulated then are much the same as the reports in circulation now, and the character given to its climate at that time unhappily clings to it still.

The second point next in order to be considered is the reason why malarial fevers figure so largely among the prevailing diseases. It will be remembered that the tables Nos. 3 and 4 in the preceding chapter give the following results. The two great medical hospitals received during 1877 a total number of 21,634 patients, of which 13,043 were due to malaria, or two-thirds of the total admissions for the year. Of course, this high figure does not necessarily represent the number of individuals, for the same patients might return more than once for treatment, and each time would be entered on the register as a new case. The years also vary considerably, and 1877 happened to be a very bad one for malaria. However, though these are very high figures, it is comforting to know that the death rate is not so alarming. A large number of the malarial fevers which appear in the Roman statistics occur, not among its own legitimate population, but among a large floating portion which lives under the most unsanitary conditions, being badly housed, badly fed, and scarcely covered by the rags which hardly hang together upon their sickly-looking bodies. These are the peasants who, leaving their homes in the healthy regions of the Abruzzi, the Alban, Sabine and Tuscan hills, come to work on the Campagna in the capacity of shepherds, or as ordinary farm labourers. Their average number is calculated as 42,000 annually, and nothing more miserable can well be imagined than the wretched existence which these poor people have. Toiling all day under a tropical sun, exposed to the wild storms which sweep over the Campagna, insufficiently housed from the bitter cold at night which succeeds the great heat by day, fed on the coarsest and most unnourishing of food, and barely clad, these labourers fall easy victims to the malaria which surrounds them, and it was from this class that the largest proportion of patients in table No. 3 was drawn. Within the city itself, at certain seasons, malarial fevers do certainly prevail amongst the poorer classes; nor is this surprising when we take into consideration the conditions under which many of these poor people live. Inhabiting districts where the poison is known to exist, the poverty and destitution which prevail render them an easy prey to its influence. From an inquiry conducted by Dr. E. Sernicoli, it was found that there were numerous underground dwellings in some parts of the new as well as in the ancient quarters of the city, many of them bordering upon close court yards, to which the rays of the sun never reach, and inhabited by the *cicoriari* (costermongers), who keep in their lodgings the vegetables and fruits which they hawk about for sale. There were sometimes as many as ten, fifteen, and even twenty persons living in two rooms, each of which was not ten feet square. One room, 40 feet long, 14 feet wide, and 10 feet high, Dr. Sernicoli found occupied by no fewer than twenty persons. In one month alone the Local Board of Health evicted 300 persons from their dwellings, and in the course of their visits, the agents of the Board found that in the Via Mesalana, fifty mud huts 10 feet wide by 8 feet high, had been put together, and that four or five persons were living in each of these, without distinction of age or sex.

Among the Jews in some parts of the Ghetto a similar, though not quite so serious a condition of matters exists, and in consequence malarial fevers are very common, in some of their severer forms. Notwithstanding this, however, the mortality from these fevers is not so alarming as might be expected. It will be sufficient for my present purpose to give the rate of mortality for two or three recent years. Since Rome became the capital the addition to its population cannot be much less than 100,000 persons. At the time of the Italian occupation in—
1870 it was 220,532, and rapidly increased as under.
1875 „ 259,290.
1880 „ .300,000.
1883 „ 310,000.

During a period of four years and eight months, *i.e.*, for 1877–8–9, 1882, and the first eight months of 1883, the number of deaths from malarial fevers was—

    1877 326 deaths
    1878 294 „
    1879 481 „ making a total of 1,101 for these three years, of whom 712 were re-

sidents, and 389 non-residents; 384 of the total number coming from the Campagna.

1882—298 cases; 222 being residents, and 76 non-residents.

1883 (till the end of August)—232 cases, 171 being residents, and 61 non-residents.

Several competent Italian authorities cast some doubt upon the accuracy of these numbers, and incline to the belief that a portion of the cases certified as due to malaria may be due to other causes, and more particularly is this supposed to be the case in regard to deaths occurring in midwinter. That these authorities have good ground for their position the following case, which I saw in consultation in January last proves. E. M., aged nine months, suffering from acute bronchitis was visited by me on the 15th of January, a hopeless prognosis was given; the child died the following morning, and the death was certified as due to *Febbre perniciosa*. However, in accepting the number as stated we know the worst, and it is gratifying to note a decided diminution in the number of cases for 1882 and the first two-thirds of 1883. It is true that in 1878 the numbers were 294, while in 1882 they were increased by four, but then the increase in population has to be taken into account, and between these two years, the increase could not be less than 20,000. Several factors doubtless were at work in producing these satisfactory results, and as I have already pointed out, one year varies from another as regards the prevalence of malaria; but while this fact must not be forgotten, other facts must also be borne in mind, and with the extensive public works which are in course of execution, the building of better houses for the poor, the disappearance of vineyards and villa grounds within the city making room for substantial and well-built houses, with the deepening of the bed of the Tiber and the improvements of its banks at several of its most unhealthy points—are all telling favourably upon the health of the city, and as the great scheme for draining and cultivating the Campagna is gradually carried out, no one can predict what the results will be upon the health and general prosperity of the inhabitants both of the city and the Campagna.

One thing, however, is certain, and that is that the changes already wrought, notwithstanding dangers which are incidental to the carrying out of such great schemes, have produced satisfactory results upon the health of the population; and as these works proceed, a corresponding rise in the health rate of the city must take place, and will show itself more particularly in those diseases which are due to malaria, and which now not only figure so high amongst its prevalent diseases, but cause unnecessary alarm in the minds of the visitors, who to only a limited degree are liable to be affected by them. Regarding the prevalence of acute diseases of the lungs, only a single word need be said. Indirectly due in large measure to malaria, which so completely undermines the constitutions of the poor by inducing chronic changes in the blood, in the liver, spleen, and other organs, as evidenced by the marked bloodless appearance which so many of the peasants from the Campagna and the poorer inhabitants of the city present—and still further weakened by insufficient food and clothing, huddled together in cold, damp, shelterless houses, without fireplaces, and without the means to buy fuel, even if they had them, the moment the winter sets in, and especially when the faintest breath of tramontana is felt, they are cut down by inflammation of the lungs and other acute chest disorders in a startling manner.

The next point for consideration, and one which more especially concerns visitors, is the important one of the mortality from typhoid fever. However, it will be readily admitted that it would be but poor comfort for them to know that typhoid fever was not fatal to the Italians, if it prevailed to a greater extent amongst strangers in Rome than elsewhere; and, therefore, I will confine myself for the moment to a consideration of its mortality among the Italians themselves, and reserve for another page the results of its effects upon the visitors, as shown by the number of deaths occurring among them. As fever, Roman fever, is the terrible threatening sword which hangs over the heads of the majority of foreigners who for a time take up their abode in Rome, I am anxious to draw special attention to this subject; and as the malarial fevers which have been already mentioned affect strangers in a comparatively small proportion, what is the fever which they so much dread, and, as one of them said to me the other day, "has cut off so many of one's friends"? This question will perhaps be more easily answered after the part which typhoid plays in the death-rate of Rome has been considered. So great have been the fears excited, and that still continue to be excited, by the mere name—Roman fever—and as the most erroneous impressions are entertained regarding it, it seems to me that, instead of going more fully into the various diseases, especially those of a zymotic nature, by which the standard of the health of a place is generally measured, it may conduce to a clearer apprehension of this important matter if I only refer to several of these very briefly, and give more space to the consideration of *fever*, by which it would appear Rome, as a winter residence, must stand or fall in the estimation of thousands in England and America, as well as throughout Europe generally.

Diphtheria has been already referred to, and perhaps, next to typhoid fever, no disease bears a closer relationship to the health of a given population, as affected by its sanitary condition. The mortality was shown to be high, but from the fact of several other diseases being included under this one term, the probability is that the number of cases of genuine diphtheria is really less than that given by the statistical bureau. Small-pox appears at recurring intervals, as somewhat severe epidemics, and must continue to do so till a proper compulsory Vaccination Act is passed by the Government and strictly put in force. In the ten years from 1871 till 1880 2,745 persons died from the disease in Rome. On the other hand, scarlatina, measles, and whooping-cough not only occur less frequently than in England, but also in a very much milder form. Regarding the mortality from typhoid fever, an important fact has to be borne in mind—viz., the large element in the population of persons who cannot, in a strict sense, be said to belong to the city at all. This element is drawn from the labourers who live in the Campagna and the annual influx of visitors, which together cannot be much under 84,000 persons; as also a portion of the great number of artisans who have flocked to Rome in the hope of finding remunerative employment and who are not registered as citizens. The Roman authorities have been in the habit of deducting a certain number of deaths on account of this floating portion of the population; and though there are good grounds for some allowance being made for the reason stated, yet an unfavourable impression is produced by it, and any such manipulation of the statistics naturally leads to want of confidence in them. The following figures include *all* the deaths from typhoid for the periods stated below :—

Year.	Deaths.	Year.	Deaths.
1875	238	1880	193
1876	182	1881	153
1877	159	1882	122
1878	170	1883	132
1879	136	1884	114*

In the first of these years the population was 259,290, and in the last it cannot be less than 300,000,

---

* Compare these figures with the deaths from typhoid fever in Paris for the same period. (*Vide* page 72.)

or, in other words, the population has increased since 1875 to the extent of about 41,000 persons. In 1875 there were 36 deaths from all causes out of every 1,000 living, and in 1884 there were a little less than 24, or about 12 deaths less per 1,000 in 1884 than in 1875, or a saving of nearly 3,600 lives in the former more than in the latter year. The mortality from typhoid in 1875 was 238, or 1 to every 1,089 living. In 1880 it was 193, or 1 to every 1,570 persons living, and in 1884 the numbers were 114, or 1 death to about every 2,631 living.

In London, out of every 100 deaths from all causes a proportion of about 1 is due to typhoid fever, whereas in Rome the proportion is nearly 2; but, although higher than London, no other capital in Europe can show a lower death-rate from typhoid than Rome. Then as regards other cities in Italy, the following table shows that Rome occupies the first place in having the lowest mortality from typhoid. The figures are taken for the years 1881 and 1882:—

Palermo . . 1·41 deaths to every 1,000 living persons.
Milan . . . 1·04 ,, ,, ,, ,,
Florence . . 0·89 ,, ,, ,, ,,
Naples. . . 0·78 ,, ,, ,, ,,
Venice . . 0·66 ,, ,, ,, ,,
Rome. . . 0·47 ,, ,, ,, ,,

As compared with Rome, no other large city in

Italy has anything like the immunity from typhoid mortality which she enjoys. Florence is nearly double, and Palermo two-thirds more than that of Rome, so that throughout Italy the fever which of all others is dreaded by travellers is found to cause a much larger proportion of deaths than it does in Rome, while among the great cities of Europe generally Rome occupies a place equal, if not superior, to any of them in the comparatively small number of deaths from this dangerous malady which occur within her walls. Moreover, while this is true of the native population, it is none the less striking when we consider the actual mortality from this cause amongst visitors. The number of strangers who come to Rome every year is reckoned at about 42,000, and of these probably not less than 18,000 are English and American. It is, of course, impossible to ascertain the exact number belonging to these two nationalities. It has been estimated by some at 25,000, and by others at 20,000, the latter being, in all likelihood, nearer the truth than the former; but even this number seems to me too high, and to be within the mark I have based my calculation upon an average number of 18,000 instead. In the case of English and American visitors, as well as Protestants of other nations, it is a comparatively easy matter to ascertain the total number of deaths occurring among them, as in every case of death, whether the person is buried in Rome or taken elsewhere, the body is in almost every instance conveyed to the Protestant cemetery and registered at the Capitol.* For the seven years from the 1st Oct., 1876, to 1st July, 1883, the total number of deaths registered was 109, or an average of less than 16 deaths per annum out of a population numbering at least 18,000. Of these 109 deaths, malaria caused 2, diphtheria 1, small-pox 2, and typhoid fever 21. The majority of the remainder were due to affections of the heart and lungs or other ordinary ailments which prevail in all communities. Therefore the mortality from malaria among the classes of strangers above referred to residing in or visiting Rome is almost nothing, being only two cases in seven years. The same can also be said of small-pox, while from diphtheria only one death was entered for the same period, and scarlatina does not appear at all. The number of deaths from typhoid fever is by no means so favourable, and has a different significance. The

---

* In the case of Roman Catholics belonging to these nationalities, it is difficult to ascertain the exact numbers, but they are so small as to influence the statistics in only a very limited degree.

total number of deaths from this cause during the period under consideration does not certainly seem high, being only 21 out of an average population of 126,000, or one death to every 6,000 living; but when we compare the number of deaths from typhoid fever with the total number from all causes it reaches the high figure of 19 per cent. of the whole. These figures, at first sight, are not a little disquieting, and were it not for the fact that the total number is so small, they would give cause for the gravest anxiety; even as it is they require attentive consideration. As has been previously mentioned, the average number of deaths from typhoid among the fixed population of Rome is about 2 per cent. of the total deaths, thus indicating for the city generally a proportion which compares favourably with other continental cities, and the number of deaths from this cause to every 1,000 living is lower than in any other large town in Italy. The typhoid mortality, therefore, is seen to press most heavily upon the non-resident population, as it is among them that this comparatively high rate is found. It has been said that no case of typhoid has proved fatal among strangers occupying private dwellings in Rome during these seven years, and that they have all happened in hotels or pensions; but this is nonsense, as within the past three years several deaths have occurred in private dwelling-houses. That a very large portion of them should be in hotels is but natural. The generally-received opinion now is that the germs of this fever are most abundant in decomposing sewage, and from thence find their way into the air, water, milk, &c.

In Rome the wells which existed till last year have been closed and built up by an order of the Municipality, and, as the water supply from the aqueducts is one of the purest and most abundant in Europe, though even here there is an element of danger, and more especially in the case of the Trevi water, which is in such requisition among foreigners as a drinking water. Yet the danger from this source is not to be compared with that arising from the unsanitary arrangements which exist in many parts of the city. The house drains are often of bad construction, being generally built of bricks or porous tufa, without a proper coating of cement, and their connections with the public sewers are neither properly trapped nor ventilated, and, what is of equal importance, the water supply to the dwellings is so arranged, frequently for the sake of economy, as to render its contamination certain.

The same cistern, often itself uncovered, is made

to supply water for drinking and for the closet, while the waste and overflow pipes of sinks and baths are made to open into the closet pipes, and even where the closet itself is trapped and flushed there is often a small sink or lavatory basin in the closet opening into the soil pipe without any trap whatever. To this latter cause—viz., the escape of sewer gas through an untrapped lavatory basin opening into a closet, no fewer than six cases of typhoid within a month came under my own notice. In this case the closet itself was a good English one, having an abundant supply of water, from which no smell could be detected, but from a small lavatory basin situated above, and on one side of the closet seat, which flowed directly into the soil pipe, came a strong sickly odour. Of fifteen persons who were known to have used this closet six were affected by typhoid. Two of these I attended in Rome; a third took ill a day or two after arriving in Florence; a fourth at Lugano; a fifth at Vevey, and the last in London. Before leaving Rome two of them complained of feeling unwell and at once left—the one going to Florence, the other to Lugano. Of the other two there could not be any reasonable doubt that their illnesses arose from the same source, although they were not laid down till the one had reached Switzerland and the other England. Happily not one of these cases proved fatal; but with such an experience as this, coupled with the fact that the disease which proves more fatal than any other to foreign residents in Rome, even though the number of deaths is so small —only three during the whole season—one can readily see why, in spite of a diminishing death-rate and an improved sanitary condition of the city generally, the old reputation for unhealthiness should still be urged against it, especially by those who have only an imperfect acquaintance with the facts. I have stated, as far as I have been able to gather them from statistics and otherwise, the real facts of the case, and if any error has been made, it certainly does not lie in the direction of favouring Rome. In its present transition state, as well as in conditions in its surroundings peculiar to itself, allowances might well have been made in several of the items in the statistical tables of her death rate; but this has not been done. There has been no manipulation whatever, and even when the whole truth has been told, Rome has no reason to be ashamed of the facts which she is able to present in evidence of her claim to be considered a city of average healthiness. There are defects in her drainage, both public and private, as well as in some portion of her truly magnificent water supply; but compare these with similar defects in other great cities of the continent, and the position of Rome will be found to be second to none. However, while this is true, there are defects which require immediate attention, and this is admitted by no one more readily than by the Italians themselves. It is satisfactory, therefore, to know that the Government and the municipality are not only carrying out with a vigorous hand the vast improvements and other sanitary works previously referred to, but that hotel keepers and householders are also fully alive to what is necessary to be done in order to make their houses as healthy as possible, and much of what has been complained of has already been remedied, and in no instance have I known either hotel keeper or householder show the slightest unwillingness to carry out any suggestion likely to improve the sanitary condition of their houses. There can be little doubt, therefore, that in the future the present small number of deaths from typhoid fever will undergo further diminution. If pure water, good drains, and healthy arrangements can destroy the power of typhoid fever, then one can look forward to the future of Rome as a healthy winter resort with no little confidence.

CHAPTER IV.

Roman Fever—Subcontinued Typhoid—Experience of Roman Fever in Florence—Quinine in Roman Fever—Cases of Roman Fever—Experience in Rome—Infective Malaria—True Nature of Roman Fever—The Roman Campagna—Nature of Malaria—Malaria at Sea—A Damp Bedroom—Bacillus Malariæ—Modes of Entrance into Human Body—Life History of Malarial Parasite—Effects of Water upon—Conveyed by Water.

IN the previous chapter I have briefly referred to malarial and typhoid fevers, and the extent to which visitors are affected by them. Although the former was found to prevail to a large extent among the Italians, and the latter to influence in no inconsiderable degree the foreigners resident in Rome, yet it is neither simple malarial fever, nor even typhoid, that is everywhere talked about, but another supposed fever which is the main cause of all the vituperation to which Rome has been subjected, which has produced the deepest impression upon the minds of travellers from all lands, and is feared as much to-day as it was several centuries ago. This fever is known by the name of Roman fever, a term sufficiently clear and definite to thousands of visitors to whom it is the expression of the greatest danger to which they can be exposed during their sojourn in the city. A name fraught with such dread, and a disease so deadly as Roman fever is believed to be, cannot be passed lightly over in any attempt to draw attention to Rome as a winter city suited to invalids, or to those to whom the treasures it contains are attractions so great as to make them willing to run any risk that they might gratify their desire of visiting a city which has played such an important part in the history of the world. The ordinary fevers best known to Italians are those of undoubted malarial origin, such as simple intermittent agues, remittent and pernicious remittent or perniciosa, while the fever equally well known to continental travellers is typhoid. Not only do the Romans know of the existence of these several forms of malarial fevers, but they are so firmly convinced of a feverish element in the atmosphere that the most trifling ailment is apt to be designated by the name—*febbre*. Indeed, what in England or America is generally called a *feverish cold*, would in Rome be styled a fever; and this is no doubt due to the fact that a vast number of Romans do suffer from malarious affections, such as the fevers above mentioned, as well as many other ailments of a more trifling nature, so that with them malaria and fever are equivalent terms, and not only so, but as I have just stated, any slight illness accompanied by the merest rise of temperature is at once viewed with apprehension and believed to be a veritable fever. The Dea Febris would doubtless be as great a favourite among the godesses with the Romans of to-day as she was with the Romans of old. The fever, on the other hand, which is best known to travellers on the continent, is typhoid, and though they may have some idea of its dangerous character, yet it appears to exercise very little influence upon their movements compared with what the dreaded Roman fever does. Very few persons, for instance, would be deterred from going to Paris on account of typhoid fever, although its reputation in this respect is decidedly worse than that of Rome; and this is all the more unaccountable when we know that the deaths occurring among visitors in Rome caused by fever are mainly due, not to some unknown fever peculiar to Rome, but to typhoid fever itself. It will be remembered that of the 109 deaths occurring among foreigners during a period of seven years, twenty-one were due to typhoid, while only two were caused by malaria. Therefore out of a total number of twenty-three deaths caused by fever among strangers dwelling in Rome, not one is certified as due to the terrible malady so widely known as Roman fever; and as the term does not appear in the mortality statistics of the Italians themselves, it must strike every candid reader as being remarkable that a disease so widely known and so greatly dreaded among foreigners should not appear at all in the statistics of the city. The whole matter seems shrouded in mystery. Strangers from almost every nation are said to fall victims to a deadly fever within her walls, and yet no notice is taken of the destroyer in the health reports of the city, and when visitors are informed that in reality no such disease is known, that a fever worthy of being christened with the name of Rome has no existence whatever, they generally give an incredulous smile at the apparent attempt to hide from them the real truth, and leave Rome more than ever convinced that something is very radically wrong. They repeat all they have heard, and, adding their own suspicions, the mystery is thus perpetuated, and the belief in a fever existing only at Rome to which most deadly effects are attributed, is increased wherever these vague reports are circulated. In this matter, as in that of the supposed great prevalence of typhoid in Rome, there is *some* ground for the belief that a fever does exist there which is neither malarial in any of its more commonly recognised forms, nor does it manifest all the symptoms which are peculiar to typhoid, but exhibits features pertaining to both these fevers, and therefore may have a relation to the one as well as to the other; but while this is the case, the disease is not by any means peculiar to Rome; indeed, the first important notice of it which we have comes from America, and among Italians no one has written more ably on the subject than Professor Baccelli, of Rome, by whom the fever has been designated *Subcontinuous typhoid.* Objection has been taken to this term on the ground that the fever does not present any of the well-marked features characteristic of typhoid fever, or of that adynamic condition known as the typhoid state. The name is perhaps not the most suitable one that might have been chosen by the distinguished Roman professor, more especially as he does not consider the fever to be due to a combination of malarial and typhoid poisons, but clearly states, in his able description of the disease, the belief that it is caused by malaria, although several of the symptoms bear a close resemblance to some typhoid cases. There can be little doubt that these latter symptoms are frequently such as might well make it easy for the case to be mistaken for one of true typhoid—in fact, it is probable that this mistake is often made; but there are many reasons for regarding this fever as being essentially of malarial origin, although presenting symptoms very unlike the recognised forms of fever the result of this poison. That there are cases of a mixed character due to a combination of the malarial and typhoid poisons is certain; but the fever under consideration does not belong to this class, and is evidently the product of malaria alone, although the poison or organism which, under certain conditions, produces a simple intermittent or remittent fever may, under other circumstances or in the course of subsequent development, be capable of producing a disease of a severer type than that usually observed as originating in malaria; that, in fact, the organism by means of a process of evolution acquires properties of a more infective nature, rendering it capable of producing results of a more dangerous character; otherwise how can we explain the occurrence of simple ague in one person, and *perniciosa* in another, both due to malaria and both alike curable by quinine? That the so-called *subcontinuous typhoid* is in this way produced I am strongly inclined to believe, and that certain cases are caused by the inception of the poison in this more highly infective form, while others are due to the further development of the poisons within the human body, receives the strongest proof from clinical experience. During the earlier years of my residence in Florence I was not a little puzzled in meeting with a type of fever which was new to me, and appeared very like typhoid, although differing from it in several important particulars; but the resemblance was so close in many of the cases that it was a difficult matter to say whether the illness belonged to the type of fever referred to, or was one of genuine typhoid. In the course of eleven years a large number of these cases came under my observation, the majority of them occurring during the spring and early summer, just the season when travellers were returning northwards after having spent the winter in the south. There was a striking similarity in the accounts given by patients as to the manner in which their attacks respectively originated. Some, after a shorter or longer period devoted to sight-seeing in Rome or Naples, began to feel fatigued and ill, this condition being soon followed by an attack of diarrhœa. Others attributed their illness to a chill, caught on their return homewards about sunset. While yet another class seemed to think the cause lay in exposure during cold wet weather while visiting Pompeii or Vesuvius; the Forum, or the Palace of the Cæsars. Alarmed lest these premonitory symptoms might develop into a dreaded fever, their only safety seemed to lie in their getting away from the spot where they were taken ill, and they once more breathed freely when Rome was left behind, and they were fairly on their way to the more northerly cities of Tuscany and Piedmont. Frequently, either from choice or necessity, a halt was made at some point on the railway between Rome and Florence, either at Perugia, Assisi, or Siena. For a day or two the change of air appeared to justify their sanguine hopes of being quite well as soon as they reached one or other of these places; but such expectations were soon disappointed by a return of the old symptoms—headache, lassitude, and a feeling of utter weariness, which continued to increase till Florence was reached, where they found themselves completely unable to proceed further, and the disease gradually developed into a more or less severe attack of fever. I observed that the longer the period which had been allowed to escape between the invasion of the illness and the patient coming under treatment the more severe was the attack likely to prove, and the more readily did symptoms of an adynamic character manifest themselves, as if, indeed, as has been already suggested, the original cause of the illness had found favouring circumstances in the body by which it assumed new infective properties capable of producing a disease not only of a severer form, but also presenting features differing from those usually seen to result from the inception of the poison in its original and less grave form. In several of the cases in which a shorter period had elapsed since the invasion, the fever showed a well marked intermittent type, there being generally two intermissions in the twenty-four hours. The temperature pursued a very irregular course, and after a day or two the intermissions became less marked, and the case gradually assumed a continued type, although frequently the temperature was higher in the morning than in the evening. In a few of the cases where the intermissions were tolerably decided, quinine in large doses produced beneficial results, but its administration was often a matter of difficulty, owing to its liability to bring on nausea or cause severe headache. The earlier in the course of the disease in which the drug could be given, it was not only more easily tolerated, but as a rule its therapeutic effects were sooner manifested, and several of the cases yielded to its influence. However, only a very small number of them reached Florence in time to give much hope that they would yield to the action of quinine. The following three cases are selected from a large number which came under my care in Florence during a period of nearly twelve years. T. M., an English gentleman, aged thirty, had spent three months in Naples and Rome, during which time he had enjoyed excellent health. On the 11th of April, 1877, he paid a visit to Frascati, Tusculum and Montecavo, returning to Rome in the evening. The day had been very hot, and about sundown the temperature suddenly fell, and not having an overcoat he felt very chilly during the last hour of the journey. On reaching his hotel he had a decided fit of shivering, and passed a very restless night. Next morning he left for Perugia, coming on to Florence on the following day, where I saw him the same evening. He complained of severe headache and sickness, and had had a disturbed motion of the bowels on the journey. The temperature was 98·8° Fahr., and pulse 86, with a dry, furred tongue and considerable tenderness over the region of the liver. I immediately gave him 5 grains of calomel, to be followed by a saline aperient in the early morning. Next day he had less headache, but his temperature had risen two degrees, and about midday he complained of being chilly. At 2 o'clock his temperature was 102° Fahr.; when I again saw him at 4 o'clock he was bathed in perspiration, but the temperature still marked 101° Fahr. Sulphate of quinine was now given in combination with salines, and the case ran the following course :—

	Temp. 8 A.M.	Temp. 2 P.M.	Temp. 10 P.M.	Temp. 2 A.M.	Quinine administered in prev. 24 hr.
Apr. 13	100·8° F.	102·0° F.	100·2° F.	—	10 grains.
,, 14	100·4° ,,	102·6° ,,	101·1° ,,	103·0° F.	15 ,,
,, 15	100·4° ,,	102·8° ,,	100·0° ,,	102·9° ,,	20 ,,
,, 16	100·3° ,,	101·2° ,,	100·0° ,,	101·4° ,,	20 ,,
,, 17	99·0° ,,	99·8° ,,	99·2° ,,	100·2° ,,	20 ,,
,, 18	98·0° ,,	98·6° ,,	98·7° ,,	99·1° ,,	15 ,,
,, 19	97·9° ,,	100·1° ,,	98·0° ,,	98·4° ,,	10 ,,
,, 20	98·0° ,,	99·8° ,,	98·2° ,,	98·0° ,,	5 ,,

The diarrhœa was scarcely worth mentioning, never more than three motions in twenty-four hours, and that only during the first day or two. There was enlargement of liver and spleen, but no meteorism, and on the 22nd of April the patient was able to take a drive. Two years afterwards I saw this gentleman in Florence, when he told me that he had had no return whatever of any symptom of a malarious or feverish nature.

The next case was a more severe one. H. E., an American lady, aged forty-eight, passed the winter months at Naples, La Cava and Salerno; returning to Naples in the beginning of May, she visited Pompeii, where she spent the day, sketching among the ruins. Before leaving, a thunder storm came on, and on her way back to Naples she felt, to use her own words, " a chill running down her back, as if she had taken a cold." Immediately on her return she took a warm bath, and had a tolerably good night. Next day she complained of headache and diarrhœa, the latter being somewhat severe. A couple of days' rest, however, and attention to her diet, seemed to restore her to her usual health, and enabled her to proceed to Rome, where she spent four days, the greater part of this time being devoted to visiting the Forum and the Colosseum. When lingering at a somewhat late hour on one of the upper tiers of the Colosseum, she had a distinct return of the " cold feeling down the back," but she walked home instead of driving, and the chill passed off. On the eighth day after, being exposed to the thunderstorm at Pompeii she arrived in Florence. On the journey she vomited a basin of soup which she had taken at Chiusi, and when she reached Florence had a sharp attack of diarrhœa. I visited her early next morning, and found her complaining of headache and nausea, with a dry brown tongue and a temperature of 101° Fahr.

The temperature for five days was as follows:—

	8 A.M.	2 P.M.	5 P.M.	2 A.M.
1	101·0° Fahr.	103·0° Fahr.	101·2° Fahr.	104·0° Fahr.
2	101·2° „	104·5° „	101·4° „	104·6° „
3	101·3° „	104·6° „	101·4° „	104·8° „
4	101·2° „	104·5° „	101·3° „	104·7° „
5	101·4° „	104·2° „	101·4° „	104·8° „

Quinine was given in full doses without producing any appreciable lasting effect upon the fever, and as the physiological action of the alkaloid was beginning to show itself the drug was discontinued. The disease now assumed a more continued form, as will be seen from the following note of the temperature.

	8 A.M.	2 P.M.	10 P.M.	2 A.M.
6	102·2° Fahr.	102·1° Fahr.	103·8° Fahr.	102·1° Fahr.
7	101·9° „	102·0° „	103·9° „	101·2° „
8	102·0° „	101·9° „	104·0° „	101·2° „
9	101·8° „	102·0° „	103·6° „	101·4° „
10	101·9° „	102·1° „	103·4° „	101·6° „
11	101·7° „	101·9° „	103·7° „	102·0° „
12	101·5° „	101·7° „	103·4° „	101·8° „
13	101·2° „	101·4° „	103·0° „	101·3° „
14	100·6° „	101·7° „	102·4° „	100·9° „
15	99·8° „	101·6° „	101·0° „	101·0° „
16	98·7° „	101·0° „	100·0° „	99·4° „
17	98·4° „	99·0° „	99·2° „	98·7° „
18	98·1° „	98·2° „	98·5° „	98·1° „
19	98·0° „	98·0° „	98·1° „	98·0° „

During the first three days profuse perspiration followed the exacerbation of fever at noon and midnight, but from the morning of the fourth day till the evening of the eighteenth there was no trace of moisture upon the skin. At midday on the fifteenth day, the temperature slightly rose, although it fell again in the evening. Five grains of quinine were immediately given and continued for the two following days, with the effect of bringing the temperature to the normal.

This tendency to a rise of temperature towards the close of the attack was marked in nearly all the cases, and gave a decided aspect of periodicity to the defervescence which, however, invariably yielded to quinine. Throughout this case there was more or less diarrhœa, abdominal tenderness, and meteorism. The liver was enlarged and tender, with a slight degree of jaundice, and the spleen was likewise somewhat increased in size. The third case, which I now give, presented clinical features slightly different from the other two. A. S., aged 29, a graduate of Cambridge and classical master in one of the great English schools. Accompanied by a friend, he took a run to Italy during the Easter holidays, spending a few days in Venice, Naples, and Rome. When he arrived in Florence I was asked to see him, and found him looking and feeling very ill. His temperature was 103°

Fahr., tongue covered with brown fur, and his pulse 96.

The history given by his friend was, that they had done a good deal of work in Venice and Naples, and in the latter city both had felt rather unwell, Mr. S. being attacked with sharp diarrhœa. On coming to Rome they visited the Forum once and the Vatican Gallery once, but Mr. S. took little interest in either, as he felt so weak and ill. They now decided to return to England as rapidly as possible, but on reaching Florence were compelled to break their journey. The following morning I was asked to visit him, when I found him presenting the symptoms already described. For six days the fever pursued a simple intermittent course of the quotidian type. The highest point to which the temperature rose during these six days was 103·8° Fahr. The perspiration was more profuse than in any case I had ever seen, and the bowels were slightly confined. A saline purge was administered, followed by quinine in full doses, but, no impression being made upon the temperature, it was discontinued after three days. The fever now maintained a continued course, for thirteen days longer, the morning temperature oscillating between 100° Fahr. and 101° Fahr., while the evening temperature never rose above 102° Fahr.

till within three days of the defervesence of the fever, when the morning temperature suddenly rose to 102° Fahr., the evening temperature meanwhile having fallen to below 100° Fahr. A few doses of quinine were now given, and within forty-eight hours the temperature was normal. On the eighth day the patient was slightly delirious, the bowels were now inclined to be loose, there was marked abdominal tenderness, with a great degree of meteorism. The liver and spleen were enlarged, and over the lower region of the former there was tenderness on pressure. On the twelfth day there was a severe attack of hæmorrhage from the bowels, which, however, promptly yielded to Gallic acid and enemata of iced water.

No rose spots could be detected, and no fresh complication appearing, the case went on well till the twenty-first day, when the temperature had reached the normal, and from this time convalescence was uninterrupted. The only marked clinical differences between this case and the preceding were the delirium and the intestinal hæmorrhage. In all other respects they were apparently similar, and it would have been a difficult matter to find their true place under any one of the recognized terms in our nosology.

That there were malarial elements in each of them no one can doubt, and yet they could not be said to be simple intermittent, remittent, or even *perniciosa*,—the forms of malarial fever with which we are acquainted. On the other hand, though they both presented features resembling typhoid, the course taken by the temperature and the absence of the rose-coloured spots deprived them of the main clinical features upon which the diagnosis of typhoid in the absence of a post-mortem examination must necessarily have rested.

Three years ago, when I took up my residence in Rome, I was deeply interested to meet with the same types of fever with which I had been so long familiar in the Tuscan capital. But it soon became apparent that though the cases were undoubtedly of the same nature as those I had treated in Florence, yet they were marked by some special features which I had not noticed in the others, and which were evidently due to the patient's coming under treatment immediately, or at least very shortly after the inception of the poison. The differences observed may be formulated as follows :—

1. That in the case of patients who were affected by malaria and came under treatment at once, the fever usually followed the course of a well-marked

intermittent, presenting the cold, hot, and sweating stages, with no bowel complication whatever, and yielding speedily to quinine.

2. In some cases the fever assumed a remittent course from the beginning, and, where it did so, was invariably accompanied by tenderness over the region of the liver, a more or less disturbed condition of the bowels, and later, enlargement both of liver and spleen.

It was interesting and instructive to observe the behaviour of many of these cases towards quinine, for while they were very intolerant of the drug when administered alone, they readily yielded to its influence when combined with an alkaline salt, either of potash, soda, or ammonia.

3. Another feature in these cases, although sometimes occurring also in the purely intermittent forms, is the sudden and great rise of temperature during their course, which frequently takes place without any apparent exciting cause.

This exacerbation of fever may amount to a rise of temperature of 4° or 5° Fahr. within the space of a few hours, and in every case where this occurred it was associated with a hyperæmia of the lungs, but of such a character that it appeared rather as the result than the cause.

4. When the patient had been exposed to both malarial and typhoid poisons, and when the latter predominated, the disease took essentially the form of typhoid. The following of an incipient stage of malarial by true typhoid symptoms, was in my experience more decided, and the symptoms more genuine in those cases in which quinine had been administered early, and its effects produced upon the malarial poison. In illustration of these points I have selected four cases which occurred in the course of last spring in Rome.

H. H., an English physician, aged 41, arrived in Rome towards the end of October. He had spent several years in India, but never suffered from malaria. Early in November, on returning from a walk outside one of the gates, during which he had lingered, observing some excavations which were being carried out connected with a large house in course of erection, he was conscious of a chill while on the spot; but before he reached his lodging he felt, to use his own expression, "as if he had been placed in a freezing chamber." I saw him the same evening, and advised his taking six grains of the sulphate of quinine every six hours. He passed a comfortable night, and felt as well as usual the following morning. About 11 o'clock, however, a slight headache came on and he complained of being chilly, and within an hour he was " freezing again." Gradually the chill passed off, and was succeeded by high fever—the temperature rising to 104° Fahr., and this in turn was followed by profuse perspiration, which did not, however, greatly diminish the temperature, as the thermometer stood at 103·8° Fahr., while the skin was bathed with moisture. On the morning of the third day the temperature was normal, and the patient felt perfectly well. However, at the same hour the headache and chill returned, followed by fever and perspiration as before, but in a less degree. An aperient was now given with the quinine, and on the fourth day the symptoms had almost disappeared. On the fifth day the patient was able to be out, and experienced no further trouble during the remainder of his stay.

L. C., an English gentleman, aged 49,—a devoted amateur artist. After having been in Rome for more than two months he began to have slight aguish fits. He had travelled a great deal, and had suffered from ague in Egypt. Without consulting any physician he took quinine in pretty full doses, which had the effect of stopping the fits. He continued to spend several hours every day in his studio, which was cold and damp, and situated in a locality having the reputation of being malariously affected. The attacks returned, but were not so sharply divided into cold, hot, and sweating stages; in fact, the fever had assumed a remittent or subcontinued course. At this stage I was asked to see him, and found him with a morning temperature of 101° Fahr., tenderness over the liver, slight jaundice, irritable bowels and enlarged spleen, with a thickly-furred tongue. The temperature at 10 P.M. was 102·2°, but the patient did not complain of any feeling of chilliness whatever. However, he could no longer take quinine, as it immediately caused a "blinding headache," but when the sulphate was changed for the citrate, and the latter salt given in conjunction with effervescent potash water, it could be taken without the slightest inconvenience. Under this treatment the morning temperature fell to 99·6° Fahr., and the evening to 101° Fahr., but the improvement did not last, and the fever continued for fifteen days longer, following a course very much like a mild typhoid case, but without showing any rose spots or any bowel symptoms, save an occasional slight attack of diarrhœa, and, with cold compresses and a light nourishing diet, the case terminated favourably, without any other complication arising.

The next cases are very instructive.

Mrs. D., an elderly lady, accompanied by a young friend, had spent three months in Rome, occupying an apartment in one of the healthiest parts of the city. This lady had suffered for some time from troublesome morning diarrhœa, for which I had seen her occasionally during her stay. Her young friend had arranged to join a party going to Naples, but the night before she was to have started for the South I was asked to see her. Finding her complaining of headache and a tendency to shivering, I thought it prudent to advise her not to think of accompanying the others. Next morning she was feverish, and complained of a *bruised* feeling all over her body, especially down the back and limbs. The temperature was 100·9° Fahr., and the headache had diminished. At midday she had a decided shivering fit, followed by fever and free perspiration. Sulphate of quinine was given in five-grain doses every six hours. Temperature at nine P.M., 102·3° Fahr. The day after, the morning temperature was only 99·6°, but towards noon the cold fit returned and was succeeded as before by the hot stage and then by profuse perspiration. At 9 P.M. the temperature was 101·4°. The bowels were regular and there was no tenderness over the liver, but the spleen was decidedly enlarged. On the morning of the fourth day the patient did not feel quite so well, though the temperature was only 99·7° Fahr. About one o'clock there was a return of the chill, which was speedily followed by the hot stage, but there was no perspiration. As the patient was flushed and restless I was sent for, and when I saw her at four o'clock the temperature was 104·8° Fahr., pulse 95. There was no cough, and no difficulty of breathing, indeed, there was not any symptom which might suggest any lung complication; but on examination there was marked dulness over the bases of both lungs posteriorly, but no alteration of the breath-sounds could be detected. Small doses of aconite were now combined with the quinine and veratrum ointment rubbed freely over the lungs, and in a couple of days no trace of dulness could be found. From this time the patient made a steady though somewhat slow recovery. During this illness Mrs. D. was not a little anxious, and suffered a good deal of fatigue from nursing, and at times complained of being weak and ill, until at length she was unable to leave her bed. She had all the symptoms of a severe attack of fever coming on. There was severe headache, sickness, and sore throat, while the temperature at nine A.M. was 102·6° Fahr., and at two o'clock it had risen to 103·4° Fahr., followed by profuse perspiration. For the next two days, in spite of quinine, the temperature showed scarcely any variation from that just given. During the morning of the fourth day, however, there was not the usual exacerbation, and for the following three days the highest points registered by the thermometer were between five and six o'clock P.M., when it reached 104°, 104·1°, and 104° respectively; while the lowest points registered were between seven and eight A.M., when it fell to 100·2°, 100·4°, and 100·2°. On the seventh day from the beginning of the attack no perspiration followed the fever, and the case gradually passed into a continued form. On the ninth day there was an abundant crop of rose-coloured spots, on the fourteenth day hæmorrhage from the bowels, and the patient did not begin to convalesce till the thirtieth day from the commencement of the fever.

The cases from which the foregoing have been selected clearly prove that a simple intermittent ague may, under certain circumstances, undergo a change of type and assume a more or less continued character, and that this change of type is apparently due to one or other of the following causes, or to a combination of them:—

    (*a*) Greater susceptibility of the individual to the influence of the malarial poison.

(*b*) A higher degree of virulence of the poison itself at the time of inception.

(*c*) The development of the poison within the body by which it acquires properties of a more highly infective nature capable of producing a fever exhibiting some of the principal features of typhoid.

Of these three causes probably the most important is the last, and that the resemblance to typhoid is of a more than casual nature is evident both from clinical experience and pathological changes revealed by post-mortem examinations. During the War of Secession in America the disease appeared among the Federal troops in the autumn and winter of 1861, and is thus described by Woodward from his observations in the army of the Potomac.

" In those cases in which the malarial affection predominated the disease presented itself in the form of a simple intermittent or remittent; not until after seven to ten days did the fever become continued, or the phenomena peculiar to typhoid show themselves,—diarrhœa, abdominal tenderness, meteorism, delirium, dry and brown tongue, and the like. But it happened not unfrequently that the symptoms peculiarly characteristic of typhoid were wanting, such symptoms as the diarrhœa and the rose-coloured spots, while pain in the region of the liver and a slight degree of jaundice were more frequent than in ordinary typhoid.

Many of these cases ran a favourable course, especially under large doses of quinine, but deaths were not unfrequent. Post-mortem examination showed, as a rule, only a simple catarrhal affection of the mucous membrane, with swelling and pigmentation of the solitary follicles and the Peyer's patches, and sometimes swelling of the villi in the small intestines with pigmentation at their apices. Corresponding changes occurred here and there in the large intestine. Next in order, enlargement of the spleen was often found, and congestion of the liver, with or without fatty degeneration. Histological examination of the lymphatic follicles in these cases brought to light changes, such as accumulation of lymphoid cells and sometimes their impaction in the nearest lymphatic vessels and in the connective tissue, which differed from the changes occurring in typhoid only in degree.

Again, in those cases where typhoid infection was predominant, the disease took essentially the form of typhoid, and the post-mortem examination showed in a marked manner the changes proper to that disease. But the disease in question was characterized by the marked periodicity of its course; the periodicity had often the typical intermittent character, becoming most pronounced in the defervescence and at the stage of commencing convalescence. Further, the enlargement of the liver and spleen was characteristic of malaria, and was not found in the same degree of development as in simple typhoid; and, finally, deposits of pigment (melanæmia) occurred in various tissues, as in malarial fevers."

ETIOLOGY.—There can be little doubt that while the disease under consideration exhibits decided periodic features in its initial and closing stages, especially the former, pointing to a malarial origin, it nevertheless presents during the major part of its course characteristics more akin to typhoid than to any other fever with which we are acquainted. Some of the pathological changes also are those peculiar to malaria, while others bear a striking resemblance to those produced by enteric fever. There is, therefore, some ground for the belief held by many, that the disease is of a typhoid character; in fact, a typhoid fever modified by malaria, or a malarial fever modified by typhoid. My experience, however, is opposed to such a view, for while many of the cases were certainly of a mixed character, the predominating poison sooner or later revealed itself, and frequently an obscure case was cleared up by the appearance of the spots which are pathognomonic of typhoid. On the other hand, cases which commenced as purely intermittent fevers gradually assumed a continued form, and during their course there was tenderness and fulness over the hepatic region, and frequently jaundice, enlargement of the spleen, diarrhœa, meteorism, pain on pressure over the right iliac fossa, dry brown tongue, and occasionally delirium, but never any rose-coloured spots appeared. Moreover, while in Florence a large proportion of the cases ran such a course as that just described; a very much smaller proportion did so in Rome, although, as far as one could judge, the initial stages in the one series of cases gave as much promise of developing into the severer form as in the other, and that they did not do so seemed to be sufficiently accounted for by the fact that they were placed under treatment sooner, and the further development of the poison hindered by the administration of quinine or some other antiperiodic. It seems probable, therefore, that the disease is quite distinct from both malarial and typhoid fevers, and is in fact a transformation of the former into a continued fever, presenting all the clinical features of typhoid, with the exception of the eruption, and producing pathological changes differing more in degree than in kind. This view is further strengthened by the manner in which the disease behaves towards quinine. During the intermittent stage, the symptoms yield readily to the drug, but when this stage is past, and the fever is developing into the continued form, it is neither so easily tolerated, nor are its effects so potent, although the addition of an alkali usually overcomes the former and increases the latter; but when the continued stage is fully developed the alkaloid has no more influence over the fever than it has over typhoid. As the contagion of malaria is now almost universally believed to possess specific properties, and as there is a steadily growing opinion that such specific diseases as diphtheria undergo a progressive development, there is not a little probability that the same is true also of malaria; at all events, it appears tolerably certain that simple cases of ague, if allowed to go on unchecked, assume a form which is not only more severe in itself, but is no longer amenable to the most trusted anti-malarial remedies; and moreover, while one attack of malaria gives no protection whatever, but rather predisposes to another, I have not met with any instance among visitors in which an attack of the fever under consideration was repeated, although in one case the patient had a slight attack

K

of intermittent ague on his return to Rome two years afterwards, which, however, immediately passed off with a few doses of quinine in combination with arsenic.

The modes by which the poison effects an entrance into the system.

From what has been already stated, the relation between the so-called subcontinued fever and malaria may be said to be established, and in order to ascertain the probable modes by which the human organism becomes affected by the poison, it will be necessary to inquire into the nature of malaria, and the extent to which it is diffused in and around Rome. In Italy there are two great regions which may be said to be the homes of endemic malarial disease—the plain of the Po and its tributaries, and the west coast from near La Spezia to Calabria. The second of these two great regions is the one which includes Rome and the Campagna. Starting from the marshy district lying between the mouth of the Arno and Pietra Santa, it extends to Leghorn, and beyond Volterra the district merges in the Tuscan Maremma, which reaches as far as Civita Vecchia. This plain is bounded on the east side by the Appenines, and on the west by the Mediterranean, and though for the most part dry and uncultivated, it is devastated by malaria to such an extent, that the inhabitants of some of the large towns, for example, Grossetto, have to leave the plain for two or three months during the year, and seek a refuge on the slopes of the neighbouring mountains; while all along the railway the officials try to shelter themselves by the little belts of Eucalyptus trees, which they have planted so as to encircle the station buildings. At Civita Vecchia the Roman Compagna commences, and extends as far as Terracina, a distance of nearly ninety miles, while its greatest breadth between the mountains and the sea is about twenty-seven miles. This vast plain, which has acquired such an unenviable notoriety for its deadly atmosphere, is neither barren nor unfruitful, neither is it covered, as many suppose, by stagnant water or marshes. True, there is an absence of trees over nearly the whole of the plain, but it is by no means barren, and what it is capable of producing under proper cultivation, may be seen in those portions in the immediate vicinity of the city, which are already producing magnificent crops of corn, wheat, grapes, potatoes, and other roots; and as to its marshy character, travellers who visit it, are not only surprised that there are no marshes, but that the soil is so very dry.

As to the nature of the malarial poison, all we

know of it compels us to believe that it is closely related to the processes of decomposition of organic matters, more especially vegetable matters; and as Hirsch says, "Inasmuch as the soil chiefly furnishes those matters, and principally aids their decomposition, we are led to assume that malaria is bound up with the soil in an essential degree, if not altogether unconditionally. In all decomposition, so far at least as relates to extrinsic activity, two factors come into account, the products of decomposition, which are either gaseous or solid matters, and the excitants of decomposition, whose organised nature cannot well be longer doubted." Of all the theories which have become current as to the nature of the malarial poison, I will only refer briefly to three, which receive considerable support in Italy from the supposed connection between one or other of them, and some peculiarity of atmosphere or soil. These views are:—

    a. That the disease is produced by weather influences alone.

    b. That it is due entirely to the soil.

    c. That it is essentially a disease of parasitic character.

There is a very widespread belief throughout Italy that a chill may bring on an attack of fever, hence the dread so many have of being out of doors in

Rome at sunset. Many Italians think that it is sufficient for a person to sit out of doors in the cool of the evening to ensure an attack of malarial fever, and it is an instructive fact, that in almost every instance, the cases of subcontinued fever which have occurred among strangers in Rome, the disease has usually seemed to arise directly from a chill.

In the last case but one of the seven histories previously noticed, this feature was somewhat striking. Two days before her intended departure for Naples this young lady paid a visit to some friends living in the Via Nazionale, and in order to obtain a view of the sunset, the party went up to the terrace on the roof of the house. Here she was conscious of a decided chill, but it passed off after dinner. The following afternoon the chill returned, and I was asked to see her, more for the purpose of deciding whether it was prudent for her to proceed to Naples next morning, than with the idea that she required any medical treatment. However, the case of her friend, who had not been exposed in any way to a chill, shows that another cause must be sought for, and the specific nature of malarial disease is so generally admitted, that the belief in a cause due to weather alone now receives very little support.

Another theory of a somewhat peculiar character

has been advanced by the accomplished French *savant*, Professor Colin of the Val de Grâce, so well known for his able researches on intermittent fever. In the view of this observer, malaria is the result of a power issuing from the soil, a "puissance végétative du sol," which becomes a cause of disease when the power is not exhausted by cultivated plants. "So far," he says, "from having to search in the vegetation of the marsh for the cause of the fever, I believe that it is rather in the inverse condition, in the absence of this vegetation, that one is likely to find it. In my view, indeed, the fever is caused most of all by the vegetative power of the soil whenever that power is not called into action, when it is not exhausted by plants sufficiently abundant to use it up." The residents on the Roman Campagna, and the peasants who go there for the purpose of reaping the crops, unite in their testimony as to the virulence of the malaria after the ground has been cleared; but as this virulence is not usually experienced till heavy rains have set in, the probability is, that the increase in the infective power of the poison is due to the moisture acting upon the soil, and not to the removal from its surface of the crops which had been covering it. Recent investigations into the etiology of the disease, render it probable that the specific cause of malaria is of a parasitic nature; and that a saturated alluvial or marshy soil becomes, under the influence of a high temperature, a very essential factor in its production; and this condition is found in a comparatively high degree of fitness in the Campagna around Rome, where a thin layer of decaying organic matter, principally of a vegetable nature, is found covering a substratum of porous tufa, which probably receives the infiltrating water from the not far distant hills, and, therefore, is independent for its moisture on the precipitations of rain or dew. But while this is an important factor, it is not the only one, and the *potentiality* of malaria may develop under other suitable circumstances, a striking example of which is seen in what has been termed *ship malaria*. There are numerous instances recorded in which crews of vessels at sea have been affected by malaria, which could not be referred to a previous infection on shore. The following account given by Surgeon Holden, of the American navy, of an epidemic of malaria on board a United States ship of war, is especially interesting: "After leaving the port of Norfolk (Va.), a pestilential stench from the bilge-water spread through the lower hold. No cases of sickness occurred among the crew, although some of them had to frequently enter the part of the hold containing the ship's stores, situated under the great cabin. A short time after, it became necessary to visit another store-room in the immediate neighbourhood of the bilge space, when the person who was sent found everything in it covered with mould, consisting of minute algæ of the family of Thallophytes. On the afternoon of the same day, that person sickened with ague, and in the days following more sickness occurred, but only in those who had entered the part of the hold which was still kept closed. The ship having put into Beaufort, the bilges were cleared out, and so long as the store-rooms were kept open, there was no fresh sickness, but when this regulation was afterwards disregarded, new cases showed themselves, but only among those—including Surgeon Holden himself—who had entered the room covered with mould." In connection with these facts, the following case is of some interest. Early last spring, I was asked to visit a lady living in a new house in the new part of Rome. Before seeing the patient, her husband gave me a few particulars of his wife's illness, from which it appeared that she had been suffering from a kind of feverish attack, accompanied by occasional chills. She had been in bed for several days, and the fever, which at first was supposed to be the result of a cold, was decidedly increasing. On entering the room it was almost totally dark, and there was a peculiar damp, musty odour. The patient disliking the light, the shutters had been kept closed, and on opening them, a remarkable condition of things was revealed. Nearly every article of furniture was, more or less, covered with mould, boots and shoes especially, and two leather portmanteaus which were placed upon the top of a wardrobe, when taken down were absolutely green with mould, although the room had not been shut up for more than five days. The case proved to be intermittent fever, complicated with slight bronchitis. Further inquiry brought out these additional facts. The whole family had suffered from attacks of feverishness with shivering, for which they had been taking quinine without any medical advice. The house was a new one— too new to be inhabited, and the apartment opposite had been vacated suddenly, a few weeks before, on account of an outbreak of sore throat. A closer inspection of the room showed the wall, in front of which the bed stood, to be saturated with damp, caused by a defect in the roof, although in the other rooms of the apartment boots and shoes became speedily mouldy when left unused for a day or two. These clinical experiences are in accord with some investigations which have been made into the nature of the organism giving rise to malaria.

Balestra, of Rome, published some deeply interesting experiments which he made in the Pontine Marshes, and in which he showed that, besides numerous low organisms in the water, there was one species of alga that grew with enormous rapidity when it was exposed to air and light, and whose spores could be detected in the atmosphere over the Pontine Marshes, as well as over the Roman Campagna. He took the fever himself twice after drawing deep breaths over a vessel containing marsh water so infected; and he satisfied himself also, that on the addition of sulphate of soda, arsenious acid, or sulphate of quinine, not only did the reproduction of these Algæ cease, but they and their spores underwent a change in their structure, and this led him to think that there need be no hesitation in designating these microphytes, or their spores, as a true cause, and perhaps the only cause, of malaria. Many other observers agree with the view expressed by Balestra. Klebs and Tommasi-Crudeli, on the other hand, found in the air and soil, both of the Campagna and the Pontine Marshes, a kind of bacillus in the form of rods and elongated, oval moving pores, which, when isolated and cultivated, produced the most marked malarial sickness in the animals which received them. The fever varied from the mildest to the most intense, or so-called pernicious kind—fatal in twenty-fours; the firm swelling of the spleen, and the melanæmia, which were observed at the same time, afforded further evidence of the identity of these artificially produced fevers with the malarial sickness occurring in man. The results of the inoculation of this œrobic bacillus are questioned by Sternberg, who conducted experiments with material derived from the soil of malarious localities in America, and which did not bear out the conclusions of Klebs and Tommasi-Crudeli. Sternberg says the febrile disorder had nothing of the character of human intermittent fever, and, besides, could be produced by other bacilli than those of malarious soil.

Still more important investigations have, however, lately been made by Cuboni and Marchiafava on the blood of patients suffering from the disease. They constantly found spherical mobile micro-organisms in variable number, and always in the interior of the white corpuscles. At the commencement of a febrile paroxysm small bacilli were seen bearing a spore at each end; their length was from one to three times the diameter of a red blood globule. During the progress of the attack these bacilli lessened in number, while free spores became more abundant. Important as these observations are, their significance is lessened by the fact that the organisms are present in the blood during the apyretic stage of the disease. Independently of these discoveries by Cuboni and Marchiafava, Professor Marchand, of Gissen, had observed in blood, taken during an attack, some small refracting corpuscles exhibiting a degree of active movement; and besides these, were other small organisms consisting of two adherent corpuscles. There were also a few long, rod-shaped bodies with swollen ends, which presented very distinct movements of their own. Recently, however, still more remarkable, and if reliable, much more important observations have been made in France.

M. Laveran discovered a peculiar organism, of somewhat remarkable character, in the blood of patients suffering from the disease. This microphyte was rendered motionless, and apparently killed, by a dilute solution of quinine, a fact which, taken along with the previous observation of Balestra, seems to afford an adequate explanation of the utility of quinine in malarial diseases.

Richard, following in the line of Laveran, has carried out a number of experiments at Philipville, where malarial fevers abound. He has found the parasite described by Laveran to be invariably present in the blood of these patients, and has never seen it in that of persons suffering from other diseases. The observations which he has made on the life history of the organism, and its relation to the malady, are in several points new. The organism has a special habitat, the red corpuscle of the blood, in which it develops and which it leaves when it has arrived at a perfect stage of development. During the attack of fever, many blood globules are seen, which possess a small, perfectly round spot, but they have otherwise the normal appearance, and possess the normal elasticity. In other corpuscles the evolution of the parasite is further advanced; the clear spot is enlarged, and is encircled by small, black granules, while around it the hæmoglobin, recognizable by its greenish-yellow tint, forms a ring, which becomes narrower and narrower as the parasite increases in size. Ultimately this substance of the corpuscle is reduced to a narrow, decolorized zone, from which the hæmoglobin has disappeared. The appearance is then that of a circular element, having nearly the dimensions of a red globule, and containing an elegant "collarette" of black granulations, which is, in effect, the organism arrived at maturity.

It is provided with one or two delicate prolongations. The parasite then pierces the membrane which contains it, and escapes into the blood plasma. In several of his preparations Richard has actually seen the organism escape from the investment which remained attached to it, on one side, as an extremely delicate circle. In other cases the mobile filament alone pierced the capsule, within which the body of the organism remained enclosed. In both cases the filament begins to move, lashing the adjacent red globules. Sometimes the recurved extremity of the filament becomes entangled in a network of fibrin, and then the movement of the filament causes the body of the parasite to oscillate. At the end of an hour, sometimes less, but rarely more, the movement ceases, and, apparently, also the life of the parasite. The infected red corpuscles present conspicuous evidence of having lost their elasticity, and become viscous. This change must interfere very much with their passage through the finer capillaries, and the number of infected globules is so enormous during the attacks of fever that the total obstruction to the circulation from this cause may well be considerable. Many other phenomena of the disease—the remarkable anæmia, the action of quinine, and persistence of the infection—are all perfectly explained by these facts.

A careful study of the deeply interesting and important inquiries discussed in the preceding pages can leave little doubt in the mind as to the real nature of the malarial poison, while at the same time they suggest the probable modes by which the parasite enters the human body. The micro-organism is found in the air we breathe, and in the water we drink. Moreover, there is not wanting evidence to show that when the poison gains access to the body by the stomach, rather than by the lungs, its action is more rapid, as well as more dangerous, and this may be due to the fever-making cause being in greater quantity in the water, or, what is more likely, to it being taken up more rapidly by the circulation and carried to the spleen. The probability, therefore, is that the malarial microphytes are inhaled by the lungs and introduced in water. Regarding the former, there is, however, a greater unanimity among observers than there is as regards the latter, although there are many instances adducible which can hardly be explained on any other hypothesis. The extent to which the germs may be carried by the wind is limited to a very small range, but that they are so conveyed is a fact which no one disputes. Sometimes, however, during the prevalence of certain winds, the wind is not merely a carrier of the poison, but, by influencing the soil becomes an actual producer of it. For example, during the prevalence of the south-west sea breeze in Rome, in summer, attacks of fever are not infrequent, and a friend, who is intimately acquainted with the Vatican, tells me that invariably when this wind blows in summer, the windows are all closed, as experience has taught the occupants that it is dangerous to be exposed to its influence. This, however, is not likely to be the result of the wind coming laden with germs from afar; but being a warm wind, and moisture-laden, it calls into activity the dormant poison existing in the neighbourhoods where it is feared. As to the conveyance of the poison by drinking water, there has been a great diversity of opinion, and the controversy has been sharp. It is not my intention, however, to re-open it, but simply to state what has been my own experience of the matter as a contribution to this subject —a subject of the highest practical importance. It is agreed by many observers that when water is abundant the malarial parasite is hindered in its development, or even rendered powerless and inert. This is, moreover, in accordance with clinical facts, for it has been observed again and again that during the prevalence of malarial fevers heavy rains have caused a decided diminution in the number of cases. But this does not prove that the germs themselves, or their spores, may not be carried by the water, and so introduced into the body. Even though also the *developed* parasite might be rendered powerless in the presence of water, it does not necessarily follow that the spores will share the same fate. Any one practically acquainted with the cultivation of bacilli know, what a remarkable degree of resistance is sometimes manifested by these bodies, a resistance so great in some cases as to defy boiling.

Balestra states that he found the fever-causing microphyte in the water, and in the report of a discussion on micro-organisms, opened by Sir Joseph Lister, which took place at the annual meeting of the British Medical Association, four years ago, I find it stated that "Klebs and Tommasi-Crudeli, injected under the skin of animals water taken from malarious localities, with the result of producing intermittent fever with enlargement of the spleen." These investigations were undertaken for the purpose of showing that the microphyte which caused malarial fever by inoculation in animals was the same as that which caused the same disease in man, and if introduced in water into the system of the animal, what proof is there to show that it cannot be introduced in the same way into the human body? The question is not whether water can produce the germ, but simply whether it can convey it. There is a vast amount of accumulated evidence from natives of all warm climates, as well as medical authorities, which apparently show beyond doubt that malaria can be conveyed in this manner. Since taking up my residence in Rome, a strong suspicion has crossed my mind that this, indeed, does take place—a suspicion which was greatly strengthened by a visit which I paid to the sources of the Trevi and Marcia waters, in the month of May last, and which I will refer to in the next chapter, merely remarking here that these two well known waters take their rise in spots where malaria prevails. The following cases, which have been already referred to as Nos. 6 and 7 in the histories previously given, along with many others, have suggested to me the probability of drinking water being one of the ways by which the malarial germs might be introduced. Both cases have been already described. The young lady was exposed to a chill on a high terrace in the Via Nazionale, and developed a well-marked malarial fever. The elder lady, being an invalid, was very little out of doors—a short walk or drive in the early part of the day being her only open-air exercise. For more than six weeks she led this life, and never went to any place where there was the slightest hint of malaria existing; and unless the poison was conveyed in some way to her by her young friend, no other source outside the house could be traced as the cause of the dangerous fever by which she was attacked. Both were water-drinkers, and the fact that one was attacked by a malarial fever, and the other by typhoid, which, however, in its early stage manifested decided malarial symptoms, seemed, when taken in connection with the history of each case, to lend support to the conclusion that the water which they drank was a factor in the production of both fevers. That being exposed to a chill without the presence of the specific malarial germ, could in itself be a cause of malarial fever is now generally discredited, and the terrace, upon which no plants were growing, was not a likely place for one to pick up a malarial disease after so short a period of exposure. In the case of the elder lady it was still more difficult to trace a probable source outside the house, and the apartment was all that could be desired, for sunniness, position, and dryness, but it had one defect. In the closet used by these ladies there was a lavatory sink, from which they were conscious a faint sickly odour came. The closet itself was well trapped, and had an abundant supply of water, and they did not give much heed to the smell which came from the "simple *hand-basin;*" and thus, for several weeks, they were exposed to its influence. The elder patient, being subject to morning diarrhœa, made frequent visits to the closet, and being also in weaker health, was a more easy prey to the poison. The source of the typhoid, therefore, may be considered certain, and, as to the source of the malaria, no other one to which both patients were alike exposed could be discovered; nothing, indeed, seemed to explain the whole circumstances so well as the water they drank together. The same difficulty of accounting for attacks of malaria have occurred in many other instances, and the question requires fuller investigation. My reasons for believing that such a mode of introduction of the malarial parasite into the human body is probable, are the following:—

> *a.* That conveyance by means of drinking water of cholera germs is now believed to be a fact. The fatal case of Asiatic cholera occurring at Cardiff last August being a striking example of it. Till we have been able therefore to isolate the malarial para-

site and study its life history and modes of development, we are not in a position to be able to deny that malaria may be introduced into the human body in drinking water.

b. That Balestra found a malaria-producing alga in water capable of diffusing its spores in the air, while Klebs and Tommasi-Crudeli were able to produce fever by the inoculation of animals with water taken from a malarious soil.

c. That the subcontinued fever, or as I prefer in the present state of our knowledge to call it, typho-malarial fever, is more prevalent among strangers in Rome in comparatively mild winters, and that in cold winters it scarcely appears at all. This fact is significant. In these mild winters the *climate* of the autumn may be said to continue itself into the winter, and as the safety of the visitor has in some measure been attributed to the dormancy of the malarial parasites during the cold winter months, it is obvious that if, owing to the prevalence of mild autumn weather in winter the parasite retains a certain amount of activity, and further, if visitors living in comfortable healthy quarters within the walls need have no fear of malaria reaching them from their immediate surroundings, there must be some way by which it does reach them, since they become affected by it; and it does not appear unreasonable to suppose, after all that has been advanced regarding the habits and life history of the parasite, that it is conveyed by drinking water, and more especially when we remember that the sources of these waters are in spots where malaria exists, and where presumably the poison is active during mild winter weather. Moreover, such a view also explains the immunity from the fever experienced by strangers residing within the city during cold winters.

Of course it is impossible to say to what extent visitors are affected by it. My experience during fourteen years leads me to believe that it is not inconsiderable. One fact, however, may be affirmed, and that is, that the fever is more amenable to treatment when taken early in its course, as is evident from the fact that only two patients died from this fever in Rome during the seven years already referred to, and no more imprudent act could be committed than to rush madly away from Rome on the slightest experience of illness. Any illness would be aggravated by such a proceeding, but especially is this true of malarial diseases in which, as I have endeavoured to prove, the poison increases in virulence the longer it is left to go on unchecked. Another imprudence frequently committed by strangers, and one which leads to much needless anxiety, and sometimes danger, is the taking of quinine without proper advice. It is the experience of every practitioner in Rome that physicians are often called to see patients whose only illness is caused by the drug which they have been so trustfully taking.

CHAPTER V.

Water Supply—Early Roman Engineers—Settling Reservoirs —Curatores Aquarum—Aqua Marcia—Aqua Tepula and Julia—Aqua di Trevi—Aqua Paola and Felice—Pollution of Aqua di Trevi—Source of Aqua di Trevi—Disease Germs in Water—Organic Matters in Water—Oxygen Method — Mineral Constituents of Roman Waters — Common Salt in Trevi Water—Trevi Water at Source and in Rome—Probable Causes of Pollution—Sources of Aqua Marcia—Receiving Chamber of Aqua Marcia.

THE water supply to large populations is one of the most important subjects in connection with sanitary matters, and one upon which the health of the populations to a large extent depends. No subject has received more attention in recent years from a medical point of view, and no one is likely to yield greater benefits to the inhabitants of large cities than an abundant supply of wholesome water obtained from the purest sources. The most difficult of engineering problems are boldly undertaken in these days, and to no more important matter—alike affecting the beauty of great cities, as well as the comfort and health of their inhabitants—could engineers, sanitarians, and municipal authorities direct their most earnest attention; as is proved by the fact that during the past dry summer no little apprehension was felt in many English cities, caused by the effects which the prolonged drought was producing upon their water supply. The ancient Romans had a thorough knowledge of this subject, and they may well be called the great sanitary engineers of antiquity. Some of the most instructive and deeply interesting studies in Rome and on the Campagna are found in connection with the ruined aqueducts which were constructed, not merely to supply water to the city, but also for the purpose of irrigating the Campagna. These stupendous works have never been equalled, and though many of these ruins still existing around Rome excite the most profound impression upon travellers, yet in other lands, but more especially in the south of France and along the north coast of Africa, similar ruins exist, and alike testify to the marvellous skill possessed by these early engineers living before the days of our own era. Pure sources of water were selected, irrespective of distance, irregularity of country to be traversed, hills to be pierced or valleys to be crossed and no obstacle daunting them, these pioneers spared no pains to secure an ample supply of pure water for their cities. A magnificent and most instructive example of this is seen in the ruined Roman aqueduct at Lyons (the ancient Lugdunum), once the favourite summer residence of several of the Roman emperors, and the birthplace of Claudius, whose palace was built on the top of the hill. Having chosen the source from which they were to draw their supply, they turned it into a stone or brick channel called a specus. These channels varied somewhat in size, and were usually lined with a very hard cement called Opus Siginum. In the construction of the aqueduct the course was sometimes made to wind round the heads of valleys instead of crossing them. At other times they were taken over on arches supported on very strong piers. Hilly ground and rocks occurring in the line of the aqueduct were generally pierced. The remains of these massive channels reveal many points of great practical interest, indicating the perfect acquaintance which these builders had of all that was necessary to be carried out in order that such an undertaking might be successfully accomplished. To provide against accidents from the immense pressure within the specus, the aqueduct was made to curve slightly at intervals of about a mile, while to secure ventilation and the admission of air, *respirators* were constructed all along the aqueducts at about 80 yards from each other, and to encourage the aëration of the water irregularities were introduced in the bed of the specus. The plan adopted for the deposition of floating matter in the water was at once simple and ingenious, and besides serving this important purpose was also made use of for supplying villas on the Campagna. Settling reservoirs, called *piscinæ* and *Castellæ*, were constructed at certain points along the course of the aqueducts, remains of which are still seen scattered in and around Rome. The number of chambers in the piscinæ varied; sometimes it was twelve, at other times four. When constructed of only four compartments, two were placed above and two below, thus—

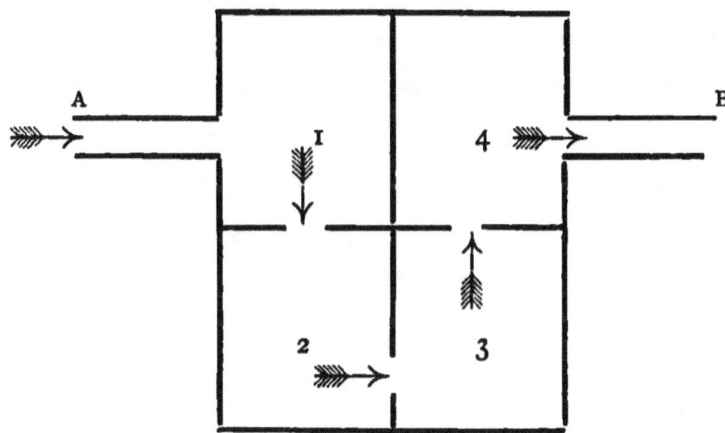

The water flowing into chamber 1 from the aqueduct A passed into chamber 2, either by apertures in the floor or by an overflow pipe; from thence it entered into chamber 3 by openings in the wall, or through a grating, and then rose through openings in the roof to chamber 4, from which it again entered the specus at B and continued its course towards the city, after having deposited a portion of its suspended matters in the two lower chambers. These chambers were so arranged as to permit of their being cleaned out when necessary. From the foundation of the city till 312 before the Christian era, the Romans had no regular water supply; they drew their water direct from the Tiber, from shallow wells or from springs—several of the latter held in honour as sacred, "for they are believed to give health to the sick." The growth of the city gradually proved that these sources were insufficient, and the construction of the first aqueduct was undertaken when Appius Claudius Crassus was consul, from whom it took the name of the Appian aqueduct. This same Claudius also made the Appian way—a road of sacred memory. From this period—*i.e.*, from 312 B.C. till A.D. 50, no fewer than nine aqueducts brought water into Rome, some of them being carried on a series of arches across the Campagna, the ruins of which are still the wonder and admiration of travellers. At first the care of the aqueducts was entrusted to the Censors and Ædiles, till the Emperors instituted the *Curatores Aquarum*, and to Augustus is due the honour of creating the new office of "Surveyor of the Aqueducts." Towards the close of the first century the celebrated general and antiquarian, Sextus Julius Frontinus, who held the office of "surveyor" under Domitian, Nerva and Trajan, and who had served under Vespasian in Britain, published his interesting work on the aqueducts and the water supply of the city. To this work and to the recent labours of Mr. Parker and Mr. Forbes I am indebted for many of the following particulars.

It is not uninteresting to observe that in after centuries, during the reigns of the earlier popes, when these aqueducts had been allowed to fall into decay, the reputation of the waters of the Tiber for drinking purposes rose so high in public esteem that Clement VII. and Paul III., upon the occasion of making somewhat distant journeys, for these days, the one to Marseilles and the other to Nice, actually took with them a supply of the water of the Tiber for their private use.

As has been already stated, Appius Claudius was the first to undertake the work of constructing a channel to bring water into the city from a distance.

Others followed his example, and the number of aqueducts constructed, varying in length from ten to sixty miles, was not less than ten, during a period of 362 years.

Frontinus gives their names and the names of their constructors in chronological order:—

B.C. 312. THE CLAUDIAN AQUEDUCT, or, as it is sometimes called, the *Acqua Appia*, was brought into the city by the Censor first named. The sources are some old quarries on the Campagna, about eight miles from Rome and a little beyond the caves of Cervara. The springs still exist, but the water is allowed to run to waste. The old *respirators* may still be traced across the Campagna, but the aqueduct itself was underground until it reached the city—a precaution necessary for these hostile times.

The Appian water was soon found to be insufficient, and in determining to augment the supply the authorities evidently had in view the desirability of having a source at a higher altitude than the springs of the Appia, and they decided upon the river Anio above the well known falls of Tivoli.

B.C. 272–264.—The second aqueduct, named the ANIO VETUS, was constructed forty years after the first, and has a length of nearly forty-three miles. It was undertaken at the request of the Senate by the Censor, Marcus Curius Dentatus. The source of this supply takes its rise on the left bank of the Anio, about twenty miles from Tivoli and some distance below the beautifully situated Sabine town of Subiaco. After supplying Tivoli, it continues its course underground to the Campagna, winding round Hadrian's Villa on its way, and reaches Rome at a point about sixty feet higher than the level of the Appian Aqueduct.

B.C. 145. AQUA MARCIA.—These two supplies were sufficient for the wants of the city for more than 120 years, for Frontinus states that 127 years after the date at which the construction of the Anio-Vetus was undertaken, that is the 608th year after the foundation of the city, the increase of the population necessitated a more ample supply of water, and the upper valley of the Anio was again chosen, and a source determined upon a few miles higher up than the point from which the preceding supply was drawn. It was no longer thought necessary to conceal the aqueduct underground during the whole length of its course, and the new one was constructed partly above ground on embankments or upon arches of masonry. Any one with Frontinus' volume in his hands can still trace with comparative ease the course of the old aqueduct from the existing remains up to the sources of the Marcia in the upper valley of the Anio, of whose excellence Pliny says, "The most celebrated water throughout the whole world, and the one to which our city gives the palm for coolness and salubrity, is that of the Marcian spring." This same water is now one of the chief supplies of Rome, and visitors may form some idea of the esteem in which it is still held by the Romans by the fact that in the early spring and summer when the countless open-air "*refreshment bars*" are opened all over the city for the supply of refreshing unintoxicating drinks, the words "*Acqua Marcia*" are invariably inscribed over the neat little tap which draws its supply direct from the main. An Anglo-Roman Company brought this water into the city the year it became the capital; and above Tivoli, a portion of the original channel was used for the purpose, but between Tivoli and Rome the aqueduct is constructed of two rows of iron pipes. It is now called Acqua Marcia-Pia, in honour of the late Pope.

B.C. 126. AQUA TEPULA.—Of this aqueduct Frontinus says, "The stream called the Tepula comes from the fields of Lucullus, in the district of Tusculum. The Tepula rises two miles to the right of the tenth milestone from Rome, and from thence is brought into the city. Mr. Forbes recognizes this source in the spring now called Fontanaccio, under Grotto Ferrata, from which it was carried underground to the arches of the Marcian, and was conveyed on them to the Monte Viminale in Rome. At various points in its course the Specus may be seen above the Aqua Marcia.

B.C. 34. AQUA JULIA.—To Agrippa, during his Ædileship, is accorded the honour of adding this to the other waters of Rome. The aqueduct is a little more than fifteen miles long from its source on the road between Frascati and Marino to the point at which it enters the city. Speaking of the Julia, Frontinus tells us that at the seventh mile on the Via Latina the Marcia, Tepula, and Julia are taken into a filtering place, where, as though breathing again after their course, they deposit mud. The two are carried on the same arcade—the highest being the Julia, the lower the Tepula, then the Marcia. Some of the most interesting ruins connected with the aqueducts are extensive remains of a great reservoir and filtering place on the Via Latina which undoubtedly belongs to the Julia, as the Specus of the Julian aqueduct can be traced to them. And on the right of the Porta Maggiore at Rome a pier in a state of good preservation is still seen carrying these channels as described by Frontinus.

B.C. 21. AQUA VIRGO.—For the supply of this water, now so well and so favourably known among visitors as the Aqua di Trevi, Rome is also indebted to Agrippa, who from the early historic notices given of him seems to have devoted considerable attention to practical matters connected with the welfare of the population. "Agrippa repaired and augmented, at his own charge, the number of the aqueducts which were so far decayed that there was scarce any such thing as water in Rome. All this Agrippa did in his Ædileship."—*Dio Cassius in Augustus.* "Agrippa in his Ædileship united to the Marcian the Virgin Aqueduct, and repaired and strengthened the channels of others."—*Pliny.*

Suetonius also tells us, that on one occasion when the people complained to Augustus of the dearness and scarcity of wine, he replied, "My son-in-law, Agrippa, has sufficiently provided for quenching your thirst by the great plenty of water with which he has supplied the city."

The account given by Frontinus is as follows:— Agrippa, after he had been Censor for the third time in the consulship of C. Sentius and Quintus Lucretius —that is, thirteen years after he had brought in the

Julia, conducted to Rome the water which collected in the meadows of Lucullus. It is called the Virgin, because the spring was pointed out by a little girl. The Virgo rises in a marshy place at the eighth mile on the Via Collatia, a wall of cement being placed around it to retain the bubbling waters which were increased by other springs. Its course is underground throughout the greater part of its length. The present supply of the Aqua di Trevi is practically the same as that now described. The water bubbles up in a beautiful little basin or valley in the Campagna, called Salone, a short distance from the caves of Cervara, already referred to. The aqueduct enters Rome under the French Academy on the Pincian Hill, after passing through the catacombs of S. Priscilla. From the reservoir under the French Academy it passes to another reservoir in the Vicolo del Bottino, off the Piazza di Spagna, and thence towards the Trevi fountain. From the Vicolo another branch passes down the Via Condotti, hence the name given to that street.

A.D. 10. The Alsietine, or Augustan, was brought in by Augustus, and was a water unfit for domestic purposes. It was chiefly used to supply the great Naumachia, made by Augustus for the representation of naval fights. The *specus* can still be traced by means of the *respirators*. About the same time also, the Emperor made an addition to the Aqua Appia, which came from the meadows of Lucullus, close to the Appian sources.

A.D. 50. AQUA CLAUDIA.

A.D. 52. AQUA ANIO NOVUS.—These two aqueducts were begun by Caligula, and finished by Claudius, because Caligula thought that seven aqueducts were scarcely sufficient for public purposes and private amusements. The sources of the former are at a lake called S. Lucia, on the Via Sublacensis, a few miles below Subiaco; the source, indeed, which is now practically that of the Marcian, while the latter was taken from the Anio, about three miles above the lake of S. Lucia, at a place called Muraccio. The two aqueducts so closely followed the same course to Rome, that it is difficult to separate the accounts of the one from the other.

Following these were many others of lesser importance, but it is necessary to refer to only two of them as being connected with the present water supply of the city. These are the Aqua Traiana and Aqua Hadriana, the former being the same as the Aqua Paola, now in use in the Trastevere, and the latter the same as the Felice, which mainly supplies the new part of Rome. The Aqua Traiana was brought to Rome by Trajan, from springs close by the Lago Bracciano. The ruined aqueduct was restored by Paul V., and is now called after him the Aqua Paola. The present supply comes from two sources. Five springs in the vicinity of the lake, with an addition from the lake itself, and after a course of about fifty-two kilometres, it reaches the Janiculum hill, where it divides into two branches, which supply the Trastevere and that portion of the city lying along the Tiber in the neighbourhood of the Ghetto. The fountains of San Pietro in Montorio, and of St. Peter's, are also supplied by it.

The Aqua Hadriana takes its rise near the castle of the Colonna, about twelve miles from Rome. In 1557 the aqueduct was repaired by Pope Sixtus V., and takes its name, Felice, from the family name of that pontiff.

Reaching the city, the aqueduct terminates at the fountain of Moses on the Quirinal, and supplies the greater part of this quarter. It is also carried to several of the other well-known fountains, as, for instance, the Triton in the Piazza Barberini, and the fountain in front of the Royal Palace.

The aqueducts at present in use in Rome are—
        The Vergine or Trevi,
        The Felice,

The Paola, and
The Marcia.

The first three are under the control of the Municipality, and the last belongs to the Anglo-Roman Company. From these four aqueducts alone, a supply of water is obtained of at least 300 gallons for each inhabitant; and when we remember that London has only a water supply of 30 gallons for each individual, and many other English cities much less, it will be readily admitted that Rome is worthy of being envied at least in one of the most important elements which together form the sanitary reputation of a great city. The four waters named are not all of the same degree of excellence—a difference due not only to the respective geological formation and other conditions affecting the sources from which they are taken, but also to the care shown in their conveyance to, and their storage within, the city. In the case of the Aqua di Trevi there is some ground for apprehension that on its way to the city it is either tampered with, or through inattention, subsoil water is allowed to percolate into the aqueduct, as there are some important differences in the analysis of the water as made at Rome and at the sources. It is not improbable that both these causes are in operation in the pollution which is now showing itself in this hitherto unsuspected and deservedly famous water. It is said in some quarters that the aqueduct has been tapped in several places in its underground course, and if such is the case, these "openings" would afford an easy means for the disposal of refuse, as well as for the entrance both of subsoil and superficial drainage waters. It is an interesting historic fact, that this is not the first time that suspicion has existed regarding this very water. Pliny, speaking of the excellency of the Virgin Waters, adds, " and yet, for this long time past, the pleasure of drinking these waters has been lost to the city, owing to the ambition and avarice of certain persons, who have turned them out of their course for the supply of their country seats, and of various places in the suburbs, to the great detriment of the public health." What the danger to the public health now is, will be seen from the thorough analysis of the four aqueducts, which was made last year under the accomplished director of the Chemical Institute of the University of Rome, at the request of the Prosyndic, Duke Leopoldo Torlonia. This important work was entrusted by the Prosyndic to Professor Stanislaus Cannizzaro, the distinguished head of the Roman Chemical Institute, who superintended the analyses;

but the practical work was carried out by Professor Francesco Mauro, and Doctors Nasini and Picini—three chemists, whose scientific work is already well-known. Nothing could exceed the care and the scientific accuracy with which the analysis was carried out; and while results have been obtained, especially in the case of the Trevi water, calculated to cause some disquietude, it is, nevertheless, a matter of congratulation that *we know* the worst, that the analysts have kept back nothing, but, with the strictest candour, have given the fullest results of their examination; and while some may be inclined to put another interpretation on several of the facts than has been put by these gentlemen, yet the analyses of the four drinking waters of Rome, presented last year to the Municipality, will compare with any water-analysis made in any country in recent times.

The Aqua di Trevi, as previously stated, rises in a small basin-shaped valley—the Valley of Salone—on the Campagna, about eight miles from Rome. So suddenly does the depression of the valley take place, that the traveller is not aware of its existence till he is almost on its edge. Before descending into it, a glance at the country around suggests the strongest impression that the valley is an extinct volcanic crater, and the waters bubbling up at the bottom of the grassy hollow are the drainage of the not far distant Alban hills. The hollow is well named the Meadows of Lucullus. Accompanied by a friend, I visited the spot towards the end of last May, and no words of mine could express the beauty of the place, covered as it was with waving fields of Indian corn, and the meadows themselves interspersed with innumerable rivulets, giving a luxuriance to their verdure, and converging to a stream of considerable dimensions, which carries their waters to the Anio which flows across the Campagna within sight of the valley. The receiving chamber is at the foot of the road by which the traveller descends from the plain of the Campagna, and within a hundred yards of it is an immense trough capable of allowing twenty cattle to drink at the same time. The hollow is occupied by a farm, and upon the occasion of our visit there were somewhat extensive buildings being erected, of a peculiar appearance, not unlike granaries in England; while lying about were immense sacks of some soft material, which one of the peasants said was *lana*. Numerous cattle were wandering about all over the valley, polluting the rivulets wherever they went. Several of the old channels were unused, and, though containing water, were cut off from the receiving chamber. One of these *specus*, which we followed up for a short distance, was overgrown with the most magnificent maiden hair fern I have ever seen. The farmer who took us round the springs told us that malaria prevailed at certain seasons, that it was sometimes very dangerous, and that all the people on the farm, at these seasons, took great precautions at sunset and sunrise, but especially the latter. To any one acquainted with the conditions under which the malarial parasite thrives, the valley of Salone would suggest the most perfect nursing ground possible—a low grassy valley covered with the richest verdure, grazed by numerous cattle which wander at will all over the place, innumerable surface rivulets which become almost, if not entirely, dry during July and August. These are just the conditions under which malaria prevails—decaying organic matters, both animal and vegetable, and a soil saturated during nine months of the year and in a semi-dry state throughout the remaining months, when the sun's rays are tropical. There can be little doubt therefore that the Trevi has its rise in a spot where malaria exists, and which presents all the conditions necessary to the production of the poison. Now as to the possibility of its being conveyed to Rome through the aqueduct.

The sources of the water are deep and perennial, for when the surface rivulets are all *drying up* the true sources become more abundant, or at least suffer no diminution; however, that they come near the surface in the hollow any one may satisfy himself. While following up one of the larger superficial rivulets, which flowed by the side of a cornfield, we came on a splendid spring of deliciously cool water, which our guide informed us never diminished even in the hottest summers. If there are therefore quantities of malarial germs in the soil and floating in the air, and if the water springs up through this soil or is exposed to the infected air, what is there to prevent the conveyance of the parasite by the water? Nor can we tell that it is there, for the methods at present employed by chemists are *powerless* to discover the presence of many disease-germs in water. The method proposed by the late Dr. Angus Smith is more promising, but until now no reliable results have been obtained.* There is another danger, however, which menaces through the water, and that is its pollution by organic matters derived from external sources. The following tables show some of the more important results obtained by Professor Cannizzaro and his coadjutors, as well as the care which

* See note, p. 188.

was taken to secure that these results should be scientifically accurate. The first table gives the dates of the examinations and the temperature of the waters, as well as the several *points* from which specimens were taken for the purposes of examination.

Water.		Date.	Temperature— Of the Water.	Of the Air.
Virgine	City . . .	28 June	15·7° C.	—
	Pantanelle	16 March	16·0°	16–17°
	Torre . .	,, ,,	15·3°	16–17°
	Junction of Sources .	,, ,,	15·5°	16–17°
Felice	City . . .	—	16·0°	—
	Sources .	23 May	14·5–15°	—
Paola	City . . .	7 March	12·2°	13·5°
	Trajan . .	29 June	17·0°	—
Marcia . City . . .		12 March	10·0°	11·5°

The next table professes to show the amount of organic matter in all the four waters, as obtained, first, by what is called the oxygen process, before the water is evaporated, and second, the amount of organic carbon and nitrogen in the residue after evaporation and combustion.

WATER.	Organic Substances.				Proportion of Carbon to Nitrogen.
	Oxygen consumed in 100,000 parts.		Frankland's Method.		
	Tidy's Method.		Organic Carbon.	Organic Nitrogen.	
	1st hour.	2nd hour.			
Trevi . .	0·0000	0·0096	0·027	0·0015	18 : 1
Felice . .	0·0032	0·0064	0·053	0·018	3 : 1
Paola . .	0·0064	0·0104	0·060	0·021	3 : 1
Marcia . .	0·0000	0·0032	0·014	0·003	5 : 1

The presence of organic matters in drinking water, as ascertained by Tidy's oxygen process, would show in the foregoing table that the Trevi water was very free from these, and this conclusion is strengthened by the aggregate proportion of organic carbon and organic nitrogen, as well as the relative amount of organic carbon to nitrogen, obtained by Frankland's process in the residue after combustion; but unfortunately implicit reliance cannot be placed upon Tidy's method for indicating the existence of organic nitrogenous matters in water. The analysts themselves admit this, as they say at page 42 of their report: "Certamente il difetto più grave del processo dell' ossigeno è di non darci alcun indizio diretto dell' esistenza delle materie organiche azotate." This is not merely a matter of opinion, but has been proved by direct experiment, and among chemists there is a very general belief that polluting materials, potent for harm, may be present in a water, the *analysis* of which would indicate it as of extraordinary organic purity. In the *Chemical News*, vol. xii. p. 24, Mr. Kingzett says: "Upon the basis of new experimental evidence, it is possible to add a certain amount of organic matter to water, after which it would pass Dr. Tidy's process as of *great organic purity*, and yet could subsequently become putrid, and therefore dangerous, in which state, judging by the sense of smell alone, or that and the use of the microscope, it would be unhesitatingly condemned by all analysts. Some time before this, I had been investigating some points in the chemical history of putrefaction, and in course thereof I had come into contact with facts which seemed to me to destroy the very ground upon which the 'oxygen process,' as defined by Dr. Tidy, rests. For instance, he says (*Journal of the Chemical Society*): 'At any rate it (the oxygen process) undoubtedly furnishes us with exact information as to the relative quantities of putrescent and easily oxidisable matters present in the water.' Now, my experiments clearly proved that the oxygen process can do nothing of the kind, for they demonstrated the fact that a water may contain at one time organic matter (extract of meat) in a non-putrescent condition, and that when these same matters—excellent food originally—shall have become pernicious, the water will absorb far less oxygen than originally. .... My experiments further showed that it is possible to introduce fifty fluid grains of a putrid extract into a gallon of chemically pure water without taking it out of Dr. Tidy's class of 'waters of great organic purity.' The putrid extract here referred to was swarming with organisms." It would seem, therefore, that little reliance can be placed upon the oxygen method for determining the presence of organic matters in water.

The method introduced by Frankland of endeavouring to ascertain the presence and amount of organic matter in water by estimating the quantity of organic carbon and organic nitrogen in the residue after combustion, yields more trustworthy evidence, and while it leaves the exact nature of the organic matter somewhat uncertain, and though in some stages of oxidation of vegetable and animal matters it is scarcely possible to distinguish by ultimate analysis between the one and the other, yet in the present state of chemical science no method gives safer indications of the freedom of water from organic impurities than this; although at the same time, in the face of evidence that excrementitious matter is finding its way into any particular water, it would not be sufficient to trust alone to the amount of organic carbon and organic nitrogen present in the residue for the purpose of determining the suitability of the water for dietetic purposes. Generally speaking, a small amount of organic carbon and organic nitrogen, with a high relative proportion of carbon to nitrogen, indicate a better water than the same quantity of these elements with a low relative proportion of carbon to nitrogen. Glancing at the table, it will be seen that the Trevi water contains more organic matter than the Marcia, but it has also a high proportion of carbon to nitrogen; while the Marcia, with a smaller absolute amount of these elements, has a less proportion of carbon; while the Paola and Felice are almost identical, and inferior in this respect to both the Marcia and the Trevi.

The following table, taken from Professor Cannizzaro's report, shows the mineral constituents of the four waters, and the differences between the total amount of their fixed constituents and the residue after being heated to 180°, to which I have added the nitrites and ammonia present in three of them.

CONSTITUENTS OF ROMAN WATERS.

100,000 grammes of Water contain grammes of—	Water.			
	Trevi.	Felice.	Paola.	Marcia.
Chloride of sodium	2·114	1·649	6·146	0·643
Carbonate of soda	4·318	2·535	2·961	0·186
Nitrate of potash	1·547	1·153	0·436	0·429
Carbonate of potash	4·586	3·337	4·223	—
Sulphate of lime	2·890	3·461	3·552	0·449
Nitrate of lime	—	—	—	0·074
Carbonate of lime	13·090	21·955	4·371	19·270
Carbonate of magnesia	3·920	5·817	3·898	6·888
Silica	4·360	4·360	1·625	0·680
Sum of inorganic fixed constituents	36·825	44·267	27·212	28·619
Fixed residue heated to 180°	36·920	43·840	27·800	28·600
Difference	−0·095	+0·427	−0·588	+0·019
Nitrites	trace.	minute trace	—	—
Ammonia	—	—	trace.	—

In addition to these there are small quantities of phosphoric acid, oxide of iron, strontium, lithium and iodine in all of them.

The above table shows great differences in the inorganic constituents of the waters. The Felice and the Marcia are decidedly hard, while the Paola is a soft water, the Trevi being intermediate between the Paola and the Marcia. The Trevi, unlike the Marcia, contains a large quantity of carbonates of potash and soda which give it a faint alkaline reaction, while the Felice, which is really a harder water than the Marcia, appears softer, from the fact that though containing a larger amount of carbonate of lime than the Marcia it also contains the same quantity of silica which the Trevi does, and after being boiled, the lime in it is apparently deposited upon the silica in the form of a fine powder, and therefore makes it really a softer water than the Marcia.

The Paola is not a good drinking water. It is not always clear, and the temperature varies, being in summer above healthy limits. It moreover contains a trace of ammonia, and is rich in chloride of sodium. From its great softness it is useful for all industrial purposes.

The Felice resembles the Trevi in many respects, and it is nearly always clear, free from odour and colour, with a pretty constant temperature of 60° Fahr. It contains little more than one half the amount of common salt found in the Trevi, as well as a minuter trace of nitrites. It may be classed, therefore, amongst very good waters for domestic use.

The Aqua di Trevi receives its name from the sources being where three ways were said to meet—

Tre Vie—Trevi. The springs have been already described. This water has been known from the earliest times as one of great excellence, a reputation which it enjoys still. It is clear, free from colour and odour, is well aërated and of a pleasant taste. The temperature is higher than the Marcia, but a little lower than the Felice. The analysis recently made suggests, however, that the aqueduct is in some way being tampered with, as there is a marked difference in the results obtained at the sources and those obtained in the city. Moreover, the amount of common salt (chloride of sodium) and nitrate of potash (saltpetre) are considerable, although the latter of these salts is not in sufficient quantity to prove hurtful. The former, however, reaches an amount beyond what some consider to be within the limits of a healthy water. It does not seem a very serious matter that a little more common salt than usual should be found in our drinking water when so much is taken in our daily food, but it derives its significance from the fact that in a large majority of cases it comes from urine or sewage. In order, therefore, to find out the probable sources of these salts, the analysts were not contented by simply examining the Aqua di Trevi itself, but they also examined two other waters, one at the Camp of Hannibal, high up on the Alban hills, and the other lower down, which supplies the village of Nemi. Both these sources are considered to be beyond the possibility of contamination with animal matter, and yet in both of them were found large quantities of nitrates, while in the former there was also nearly as much common salt as in the Trevi itself. As there is no ammonia in this water, a mere trace of nitrites and very little organic matters, the analysts express their belief that these salts must be derived from vegetable matter in the soil, or if due to contamination from animal matters, that the long filtration through such porous soil as the tufa and pozzolana of the Alban hills and Campagna present, must be a sufficient guarantee of the complete oxidation of such matters and the consequent purity of the water, an opinion shared by many other eminent chemists.

Probably, also, to the same source may be attributed the trace of nitrites which is found in the Aqua di Trevi, although there is ground for some apprehension that animal excrement is finding its way into the water in some part of its course, a fear which is further strengthened by the fact shown by the analysts—namely, that the sum total of the solid residue suffers loss when heated to 180°, and that in the analysis made at the sources and at the springs are several important differences, as the following table shows :—

Aqua de Trevi.	Residuo Solido a 180°.	Anidride Nitrica.	Nitriti.	Sostanze Organiche.	Cloro.
Citta . . .	36·92	0·826	tracce	0·017	1·283
Pantanelle . .	51·00	0·787	—	—	1·450
Torre	31·20	—	tracce minime	—	1·270
Punto d' Unione .	41·80	0·714	—	—	1·221

"Questi numeri ci dicono che le acque delle sorgenti sono anche più pure di quella che si distribuisce a Roma e ci inducono anzi a sospettare, lungo il condotto, qualche possibile filtrazione. La qual cosa viene confermata dal fatto che l'acqua giunta a Roma, ha un residuo fisso minore di quello che aveva al punto d'unione; e siccome nell' acquedotto non si forma deposito alcuno ci troviamo costretti ad ammettere (tutte le volte che la variazione non voglia attribuirsi all' averle attinte in diversa epoca) che vengono a mescolarsi dal di fuori acque un po'meno pure e mene ricche di sostanze solide. Noi non staremo ad insistere sulla gravità di questo fatto, vogliamo sperare che le acque infiltrantesi non sieno nocive e neppure sospette, ma certo non v'è garanzia per la pubblica salute se un'acqua anche di ottima qualità non venga condotta e distribuita senza che vi sia stata la menoma comunicazione coll' esterno, poichè, se anche attualmente si trova buona, nessuno può escludere che per le parti dell' acquedotto, guaste dal tempo o per quasiasi altra ragione non rispondenti allo scopo, possa un giorno o l' altro inquinarsi.

"Lo studio delle acque attinte alle sorgenti ci può spiegare forse quella certa variabilità di composizione minerale che presenta l'Acqua Vergine, e che è stata constatata da diversi sperimentatori. Si vede che mentre la purezza organica non lascia in tutte e tre le sorgenti nulla a desiderare, il residuo è assai diverso e quindi si comprende come, se la quantità d' acqua che viene dall' una varia in un dato momento respetto alle altre, la proporzione di materie solide disciolte deve necessariamente variare nell' acqua che si conduce a Roma e che senza dubbio va annoverata tra le migliori."

There is sufficient ground in this statement, taken in connection with what was previously said regarding the condition of matters at the fountain head to cause considerable disquietude. It is neither satisfactory to know that the sources are actually in a low valley, occupied by a farm, with all the possible contamination associated therewith, and where the conditions for the production of malaria are as favourable as could well be supposed, nor to be assured that there is reason to believe that the water in the aqueducts is exposed to infiltration from without, or what is probably worse still, that openings have been made into the aqueduct for the purpose of clandestinely drawing water from it, as well as to afford a ready means for the disposal of excrement. The dangers of subsoil water have been already referred to, and the close relations which exist between this cause and the prevalence of such diseases as malarial fevers, diphtheria, and typhoid, and, therefore, any such danger menacing Rome through inattention to a matter so easily remedied is to be deplored; and further, it is not a pleasant idea which is suggested by others, that the aqueduct may be now in use by some unscrupulous persons for the purpose of disposing of their sewage. It is to be hoped, therefore, that the Municipality will take immediate steps to ascertain the cause of these defects, and subject the whole course of the aqueduct to the strictest scrutiny, and thus add to the boon already conferred in calling attention to the danger, another greater still—the placing beyond doubt of the reputation of a water which has been known since the days of the Cæsars as one of the purest and pleasantest drinking waters in Europe. It is also a matter of great satisfaction to know that steps are in contemplation by the authorities for *enclosing* the springs. Of this the farmer of Salone told us, while expressing great regret at the prospect of that portion of his farm being taken from him. No true well-wisher of Rome, however, will share in this regret ; and if the measure is carried out, the valley drained to carry off speedily the surface water, and the aqueduct itself put in thorough repair, the Trevi water will be placed beyond the faintest suspicion.

Regarding the Aqua Marcia no such danger threatens as that which menaces its popular rival, the Trevi, the total amount of organic carbon and organic nitrogen being very small, although the proportion of the former to the latter is not quite so reassuring as in the case of the Trevi ; but as this varies in different waters, the relative high amount of nitrogen to carbon may have no serious meaning. It contains no potash, very little soda, and a very small quantity of nitrate of potash and common salt. It is, however, rich in carbonate of lime ; hence its hardness. The water is therefore one of extreme purity as well as coolness. At the fountain head it has a pretty constant temperature of $48\cdot2°$ Fahr., and in Rome of 51·8° Fahr. Accompanied by Mr. Forbes, whose knowledge of the old aqueducts is only equalled by his willingness to impart that knowledge to others, I made a very careful examination of the district from which the Marcian waters are drawn, and the little map on the next page, is from a sketch taken on the spot. The Lago Lucia is about seven miles below Subiaco, and skirts the old Via Sublacensis, commencing a little beyond the point where the Via Valeria turns to the left. Proceeding towards Subiaco, the great limestone rocks, from which the water takes its rise, are on the left of the road, while the Lucian lake is close to the other side, and extends beyond the Serene Waters to the Mole of Agosta. To the extreme right of the valley the Anio flows in its course towards Rome, and the ground lying between the road and the river is partly marshy and partly cultivated. The marshy portion extends along the whole length between the lake and the Mole of Agosta, and in some places is of considerable breadth. It is intersected by innumerable little streams, which gather into a larger channel or canal, and find their way into the Anio. The ground, however, is very boggy, and in many places the water is stagnant, while in others it is covered with the most luxuriant vegetation. Between the lower end of the Lucian lake and the Mole is a distance of about three miles, and is filled up by the lake, and a series of small lakes, or rather springs, which diminish in size as they ascend. The valley also narrows at its upper end, and at the bridge of Marano the Anio is on the same level as the springs, and when in flood overflows all the marshy tract lying towards the Lago Lucia. For a distance of several miles above Marano the river maintains the same high level, and the ground is composed of the *stiffest* clay I have ever seen. The ancient Claudian and Marcian waters took their rise principally in that portion of the district lying immediately between the Lago Lucia and the Aqua Serena. To the old Marcian, Caracalla added a spring from the *Aque Serene*, while Augustus brought another called *Le Rosoline* from near Agosta. It was in these same Serene waters that the Emperor Nero, according to Tacitus, added one to the many foolish things which he did during his reign. The historian says—" Nero entered for the purpose of swimming in the fountain head of the Marcian water, which is conveyed to the city. He was considered to have polluted the sacred water and to have profaned the sanctity of the place by washing his person there; and a dangerous fit of illness which followed left no doubt of the displeasure of the gods."

Over one of the old Marcian springs, close to the Aqua Serena the receiving chamber of the modern Aqua Marcia-Pia is built, while a little beyond a magnificent stream gushes from beneath the rocks, and crosses the road to Subiaco. The receiving chamber is a large room, into the centre of which one is able to enter by means of a bridge or stage rising out of the water. The day on which we visited this interesting spot was one of unusual warmth, and the delicious coolness experienced while standing over the rushing water will not soon be forgotten. Three conduits convey the water into the chamber, while another conveys it into the specus on its way to Rome. Beside this outlet there is a second which is used after stormy weather, when the water is apt to be turbid, for the purpose of allowing the turbid water to flow into the Anio. The position of the Anio is in close proximity to and capable of overflowing the spot.

Where the Marcian waters are *gathered* readily accounts for that water being sometimes turbid on its arrival in Rome. The marshy ground might easily be more thoroughly drained, and all surface water made to flow by proper channels into the

Anio, while towards Marano a little embankment would prevent any overflow from that river into the springs above the Aqua Serena. Malaria exists throughout the neighbourhood, and as we were informed on the spot, sometimes rather severely. This is an additional reason why the ground around the receiving chamber should be as far as possible protected from the risk of the superficial water contaminating the perennial stream which flows from the limestone rocks above.

NOTE (referred to on page 171).—Important experiments are being conducted with *coke, spongy iron, animal charcoal,* and other filters, with the view of testing their power of removing those micro-organisms from drinking-water whose presence could be detected by Koch's bacteriosopic method. The coke and spongy iron have yielded very promising results.

CHAPTER VI.

Precautions to be taken in Rome—Chief Dangers of Roman Climate—Cold Weather in Rome—Choice of an Apartment—Roman Habits—Acclimatization—Warm Clothing—Imprudences of Visitors—Animal Food—Sleeplessness—Sight-seeing—Exposure at Sunset.

IN a city like Rome, having a subtropical climate, subject both to sudden and great variations of temperature during the winter and spring months, there are certain precautions to be taken, and certain climatal conditions to be understood, in order that the visitor may enjoy the privileges of a winter residence without being exposed in an unnecessary manner to any risks which may be peculiar to the climate or place. One of the chief dangers of the Roman climate, is that which arises from its great variations of temperature, causing injurious effects which are likely to disturb the equilibrium in organisms exposed to them. Persons in weak health are affected by these changes more readily, and they cannot so easily compensate for the disturbance caused as more robust persons can. This danger is in proportion to the suddenness and greatness of the variations in temperature presented by any particular climate, and, as has been already pointed out, the changes in the temperature of Rome during the winter and early spring months, are both very great and take place with startling suddenness. Few visitors have any idea how severe the cold can sometimes be in Rome, and in their choice of an apartment they frequently make the mistake of underrating the importance of this fact. Beguiled by the bright sunshine, they will often decide upon a house in which many of the rooms are without fireplaces, and if they have them, they are in such inconvenient places, and of such bad construction, as to be practically of little value in warming the air of the rooms. There is no matter more important as likely to affect the comfort and health of visitors than this, and more particularly is it true in the case of elderly people with feeble circulations. It not infrequently happens, in a comparatively mild winter or spring day, that the thermometer will rapidly fall to several degrees below freezing by a sudden change in the direction of the wind, and it is during these sudden and severe changes in the weather that the dangers of improperly heated apartments are more keenly felt. Of course, it does not necessarily follow that the rooms must be warmed by stoves or fireplaces. Apartments having a southern or western exposure, with nothing to obstruct the full entrance of the sun's rays, rarely require any fire at all, and if such a residence can be secured by the visitor—and there are many of them to be had—a warm, genial, sunny day may be experienced in the house, when out of doors, in places exposed to the north wind, the thermometer may mark several degrees below freezing. On the other hand, apartments not having a warm, sunny exposure, are often colder than the streets outside; and every resident in Rome has been struck with the manner in which the Romans themselves endeavour to lessen this danger. Instead of putting on, as we do, their heaviest and warmest wraps to walk out of doors, they reserve them for their return, and on reaching home they put off their lighter wraps and put on their heavier ones; and if this is not sufficient, and they have neither stove nor fireplace, they have recourse to the *scaldino*, a little metal or porcelain brazier, which is filled with *carbonella*, and yields a considerable amount of heat. Ladies place these braziers under the chairs where they sit, or more frequently carry them about in their hands. In the coldest day in winter, a Roman matron may be seen idling her time at the open window, observing the passers-by, very insufficiently clad, but holding in her hands the little "porcelain fire-basket;" and it need not, therefore, be a matter of surprise, that bronchitis and pneumonia are common among them during the cold weather. There is a general impression among the Romans that English and American visitors make too much of this matter of warming their apartments, and believe that it is sometimes carried to an extent beyond the limits of health. This may be true in certain cases, but my experience is that the dangers lie mainly the other way, and the members of these nationalities should exercise the same judgment in the choice of an apartment in Rome, as they would do in New York or in London. It sometimes happens that rooms are heated by means of large braziers, which, if they contain *carbonella*, are harmless, but if, as is often the case, the carbonella is mixed with pure charcoal, they become highly dangerous. Last winter I attended three cases of charcoal poisoning, one of them occurring in one of the most expensive apartments in Rome. There is no peculiarity in the climate beyond the great variations already alluded to, which need be taken into account in fixing upon a residence for the winter, unless it be to avoid, for the present, those quarters where building operations are going on, necessitating the upturning of the soil, and, consequently, some little risk from malaria. The influence of what is termed *acclimatization* may be entirely left out of reckoning, indeed, the word should be expunged from our vocabulary altogether, as it has had so many meanings, and has been taken to express results and conditions which have not been borne out by observation and experience. There can be little doubt that the human body does, within certain limits, accommodate itself to variations of temperature, and that, in warm climates, the lungs act less, and the skin more, while the circulatiion is lowered; and we may conclude that the converse holds true in the case of cold northern climates, a conclusion supported by the experience of natives of warm climates taking up their residence in cold temperate countries. To this extent, therefore, there may be said to be *acclimatization*, or rather *accommodation;* but there is no evidence forthcoming to show that the usual belief is true, that the constitution in some way acquires a power of resisting unhealthy influences—a power of not being any longer susceptible to them; and, therefore, visitors intending to take up their residence in Rome, for a shorter or longer period, need have no anxiety on the point of being *unacclimatized*, beyond the precautions requisite to preserve them from unnecessary exposure to a sudden chilling of the atmosphere, and by conforming in some degree to the habits of the natives, both in dress and food. Frequently one sees patients in Rome whose illnesses have been brought on by insufficient warm clothing, and there is no city in Europe where flannel in abundance, and warm coverings of every kind are more necessary in winter, than in the Italian capital. The habits of the Romans, too, in the matter of exposure to the evening air, especially in places known to be malariously affected, should be attentively considered. They are most careful in their avoidance of those spots after sundown, and the manner in which strangers expose themselves excites the most genuine surprise among the Italians, and they cease to wonder at the reports of illness occurring amongst the visitors, when they witness the imprudences of which they are guilty—imprudences which, if committed elsewhere, would not be less dangerous in their results. During last winter an English officer, residing with his family in Rome, invited a number of friends to supper and a dance. Towards midnight a large number of the party walked to the Colosseum, where they spent a couple of hours admiring the colossal ruins in the soft moonlight, returning to their homes in the early morning. Two of them were a few days afterwards laid down with fever, a fact which will excite no surprise. In the matter of food an impression prevails among English physicians that animal food is less required in Italy than it is in England, but my experience does not bear out this impression. The better class of Italians generally, and the Romans particularly, consume a considerable quantity of animal food, as well as maccaroni, which is the nitrogenous portion of wheat without the starch. In spring and summer there is certainly less animal food taken in Italy than in England, but during the winter no such difference is, as far as my experience goes, to be observed. Hence in summer, ordinary diarrhœa in Italy is generally treated by mineral acids or lemon-juice; whereas in England alkalies are more often prescribed, a difference in treatment partly due to a difference in the kind of food used by the two nationalities. A liberal and nutritious diet is as necessary in Rome as elsewhere, and no strict rules can be given for the food to be partaken off there, which are not applicable to other places as well; beyond the fact that, possessing a subtropical climate, as Rome does, the digestive process is not so vigorous, and, therefore, animal food, in its lighter forms, should be more freely taken—a recommendation easily carried out from the plentiful supply of game, venison, and chickens, always found in the Roman market. Regarding stimulants, the more closely visitors follow the example of the Natives, both in the amount as well as in the kind of stimulant they take, the better is the climate likely to agree with them. Strong alcoholic and malt liquors are neither suitable nor necessary for the majority of strangers visiting Rome; and unless there is some special indication for their use, they had better be avoided altogether. The nervous system is much more awake to the effects of alcohol, and, therefore, less quantities are instinctively taken to produce the required effects. Very few Italians are water-drinkers, but there are very few, indeed, who are addicted to the abuse of alcohol; and no greater contrast can be seen between Italy and England than that which may be so frequently witnessed among holiday-makers in the two countries. In Italy thousands of Italians, with their families, may be seen returning from a holiday without a single case of inebriation among them, a striking contrast to what is invariably the experience in England.

Another feature apt to appear in the life of non-residents in Rome is sleeplessness, an experience, indeed, which is felt by strangers more or less throughout the whole of Italy. It does not usually continue long, nor are its effects attended by the same discomforts as they usually are in our homelands. The nervous system being more alert and active, is better able to get through the work of the day with less exhaustion from it, and, therefore, as a rule, nothing is required in the way of treatment, and certainly recourse should not be had to opium, chloral, or any similar drug, as they only increase the trouble. It is better to allow the want of sleep to be made up by an afternoon nap, until the constitution has accommodated itself to its new surroundings.

Bodily exercise is of the greatest importance, and should be taken whenever the weather is suitable. No greater mistake can be made by visitors than to spend their entire time in visiting the churches, galleries, and other *sights* of the city, as is so frequently done in Rome. Fatigue and nervous exhaustion are sure to follow, and complaints are made against the climate, and of illnesses due to it, which might be more truly laid at the door of the complainants themselves. Two winters ago, two English ladies, who had been advised by me to *winter* in Rome, came, about ten days after their arrival, complaining that they must leave at once, as they both felt convinced that the climate did not suit them. They returned, they said, from their day's sight-seeing so utterly exhausted that they were scarcely able to go upstairs to their rooms. On inquiry, I found that their whole day was devoted to visiting places within the city, while the evening was given to reading and taking notes of the day's work. The fact was that they were thoroughly overtaxed, were sleeping badly, and, at times, were so tired as scarcely to be able to take their meals, while frequently their midday meal was nothing more than a biscuit, as they could not *afford* the time to return to their hotel for lunch. They were advised to take life more easily, and devote at least two hours every day to a drive on the Campagna, in the Villa Borghese, the Pamphili Doria, Monte Mario, the Appian Way, or some other of the delightful excursions around Rome, with the result that all their *weaknesses* left them, and with them also their fears, and they spent, as they afterwards acknowledged, one of the most pleasant and profitable winters they had ever enjoyed on the Continent.

There is one danger which has taken a very deep root in the minds of nearly every visitor who has come to Rome, and that is, the danger supposed to be incurred by being out of doors at sunset, a belief which has been strengthened, and continues to be so, by the reports of fever being so easily caught at the close of the day, when the temperature is falling rapidly. Everywhere throughout Italy the same thing is stated by all who reside in districts where malaria prevails, and the statement is true, and the cause is easily explained. But it is not only at sunset that the danger is incurred—it is greater even just before, or at sunrise. Observations made in connection with the dew-fall have revealed that just at sunset a very great diminution of temperature takes place in the stratum of air lying immediately above the ground—just, in fact, the stratum which has been warmest throughout the day, and that this diminution in temperature does not only continue throughout the night, but increases immediately before sunrise. Now, it will be remembered that a chill invariably appeared to be the beginning of the malarial attacks previously described, not because a chill in itself could produce the attack of fever, but because the cold so *lowered* the vitality of the individual as to render him more susceptible to the influence of the poison. Hence the reason why sunrise is more justly dreaded by Italians than sunset. But this remark only applies to spots where malaria is known to exist, and any person, if protected by suitable precautions, such as an extra shawl or overcoat, may be unhesitatingly exposed to the air of Rome within the walls by night as well as by day without incurring any risk of fever whatever.

If visitors, therefore, would exercise ordinary prudence, and be careful not to fatigue themselves by rushing about in the manner which so many of them do, exhausting their nervous systems by overwork, and then, on their return to their hotels or lodgings, indulging too freely both in eating and drinking, disturbing their digestion and their sleep, and thus rendering themselves a more easy prey to any poison, such as typhoid or malaria, to which they may be accidentally exposed.

CHAPTER VII.

Mineral Waters in Italy—Alban and Sabine Towns—Seaside Resorts—Civita Vecchia—Palo—Porto D'Anzio—Tivoli—Subiaco—Olevano—Albano—Frascati—Rocca di Papa—Monte Cavo.

TILL within the last few years, there were very few spots throughout the whole of Italy where visitors could spend the summer months with any degree of comfort, and this, not because there were no suitable summer resorts available or within easy reach, for they are numerous enough ; but the great desideratum has been, and in some quarters still is, comfortable hotels or pensions, such as one finds scattered all over Switzerland, nestling in the most lonely unfrequented valleys, or perched on some almost inaccessible peak. Excepting Switzerland, not many countries possess more beautiful alpine and subalpine scenery, or are richer in mineral waters than Italy ; even Switzerland itself does not surpass for beauty some of the higher valleys of the Sabine country, the hills of Tuscany, or the snowy ranges at whose feet the thriving towns and villages of Piedmont lie. Nor can Germany and France boast of richer treasures in mineral springs than those found on the Italian side of the Alps, and it is therefore not surprising that many Germans frequent the famous Spa of Montecatini in preference to their own Carlsbad. The thermal Grotto of Monsummano—within a short distance of Montecatini—has a great reputation in chronic articular and other affections, and presents statistics which will bear comparison with Aix-les-Bains or Wiesbaden; while the mud baths of Acqui are not behind those of Franzensbad or Marienbad, and the waters of Chianciano produce results in cases of gout and gravel equal to those obtained at Contrexville or Vichy. But unless in a few places, such, for instance, as Montecatini, Recoaro, and Acqui, where the hotels are very comfortable, there is no accommodation at many of them; and especially at the mineral springs, where one could send patients to, as the arrangements are of the most primitive character, and are thrown completely into the shade when compared with the excellently appointed and ably conducted Swiss and German establishments. This is to be regretted, because not only are these waters invaluable for many diseased conditions, but they are easily reached by visitors who may have *wintered* in Italy, and frequently, visits could be made to them in the early summer—just the time when visitors are returning northwards, and too soon to go either to Switzerland or Germany.

The same is true of summer quarters in Italy. At present, of the many thousands who visit Italy every season, very few spend their summers in the country, although they may have the intention of returning for the winter. After Easter, Rome suddenly empties, and the streets soon become deserted. Tourists and others flock northwards, visiting Tuscany, Lombardy, and Piedmont on their way, and finally cross the Alps to find a summer resting-place in some lovely Swiss or Tyrolese nook. If suitable spots could be found on the Italian side, where visitors might pass their summer months, and where the accommodation was both comfortable and reasonable, no doubt a large proportion of those who are now compelled to leave Italy when the warm weather sets in, would remain in the country, not only saving the expense and fatigue of long railway journeys both to and fro, but they would be able to enjoy the Italian climate at two of the finest periods of the year—the early summer, and the time of the gathering of the grapes. They would see Italian scenery in its richest colours, and become acquainted with many of the charms of Italian life, which visitors to

Florence, Rome, or Venice know almost nothing of, simply because they rarely see or come in contact with it. Southern Italy, notwithstanding her many advantages, has not kept pace with her sister in the north in the development of her resources, in the opening up of summer quarters, and *Stabilmenti dei Bagni*. In Lombardy and Piedmont summer bathing establishments are springing up in all directions, and in the higher valleys lying among the mountains to the north of Milan and Turin are several of these, and though frequented by considerable numbers of Italians, are scarcely so well known to foreigners as they deserve to be. No more delightful retreat could be found for the months of May, June, and September than Billa Andorno—a beautiful spot about equidistant from Turin and Milan, situated at the entrance of the lovely valley of the Cervo, and within view of the snowy slopes, below which are the famous establishments of the *Sanctuarii*. There are very few places in the immediate vicinity of Rome suitable for this purpose at least for the present, and until considerable advance has been made in the draining and cultivating of the Campagna, with the completion of the great sanitary measures now in process of execution within the city itself, it would not be desirable for strangers to return to Rome before

October. So that while there are several beautiful spots in the neighbourhood of the city having a temperature sufficiently cool, with fairly comfortable accommodation, and abundance of shade rendering them very desirable summer resorts, yet there is no intermediate climate between these and Rome itself; and there are no spots within easy reach where visitors, leaving these retreats, could pass the time till they returned to Rome.

In the near future there is every hope that strangers may come as safely to Rome in September as they now do to Florence or Turin, or any other Italian town; and with the opening of comfortable hotels at Rocca di Papa, Albano, Frascati, Tivoli, Subiaco, and Olevano, there will be no need for any intermediate place between these and the capital, as visitors could remain at all of them till near the end of September. A more pleasant summer could scarcely be spent than a sojourn in these Sabine and Alban towns, and as they are all within easy access of each other, either by rail or good carriage roads, a series of brief visits would enable one, in turn, to know them all; and while thus enjoying a summer residence in the mountains, an opportunity would also be given of becoming acquainted with some of the most interesting historic spots in Europe, which is not too much to say of a district which contains the farm of Horace, the chief springs of the ancient as well as the modern water supply of Rome, which has witnessed many of the orgies of Nero as recorded by Tacitus, and is the cradle of the Benedictine monks. Even to-day the desolate valley which became the *rendezvous* of the disciples of St. Benedict has lost none of its savageness, while nothing can exceed the solemn grandeur of the situation of the Convent of *S. Scholastica*, dedicated to the sister of the founder of the Benedictine Order, and surrounded by the solitary peaks of the mountain chains which so closely encircle the town of Subiaco.

With the exception of Subiaco, and probably also Frascati and Albano, none of the towns within easy reach of Rome are therefore suitable as summer quarters for foreigners. However, during the spring and early summer months, they are valuable resorts, to which a run may be made from Rome either by invalids who require change of air, or by visitors who wish to escape the beginning of the warm weather in the city. The places available for this purpose, and which present the greatest attractions to strangers are Porto D'Anzio, Palo, and Civita-Vecchia by the sea. Tivoli, Subiaco, Olevano, Frascati, Albano, Nemi and Rocca di Papa, on the Sabine and Alban hills. Civita-Vecchia is about two hours from Rome, and situated on the railway to Pisa, at the point where the Tuscan Maremma merges in the Roman Campagna. Immediately opposite the station there are two large sea-bathing establishments which are greatly frequented by the Romans in summer. The season begins about the middle of June and lasts till the end of August. Between the railway station and the harbour—the old Porta Romana, built by Trajan and admirably described by Pliny—is a very fine Esplanade, which is now occupied by several massive buildings, and others are in course of erection. At the extreme end of the Esplanade overlooking the port is the Hotel Orlando, now entirely cast into the shade by the magnificent thermal establishment and hotel which is situated about the centre of the Esplanade, and is supplied by the ancient springs which were used by Trajan for his villa and thermæ. The sources are about three miles from the town, and the waters there have a temperature of 95° to 130° Fahr.

The mineral ingredients are mainly muriate and sulphate of soda, sulphate of magnesia and carbonate of lime, with a little iron and arsenic, and the temperature of the water at the thermal establishment is only a few degrees less than that of the springs. These waters have a considerable reputation in cases of chronic arthritis, gout, and scrofula, and during a recent visit which I made to this establishment I met an old naval officer, who told me that he saw Garibaldi carried into the baths a helpless cripple, and in less than a fortnight the veteran soldier was able to take his daily *constitutional* on the Esplanade. Palo is a little place, now rising into note as a seaside resort. It is about midway between Rome and Civita-Vecchia, and, like Porto D'Anzio, is visited by sportsmen in May, as the neighbourhood abounds with quail.

Another interesting place, now frequented by visitors during the early spring, is Porto D'Anzio, the representative of ancient Antium, the capital of the Volsci, and one of the most important naval stations of Imperial Rome. Porto D'Anzio reached the height of its prosperity during the decline of the Republic, and under the Empire, and was a favourite resort of the Emperors. It was here that Augustus received the title of Pater Patria, and where Caligula and Nero were born. Cicero had two villas in this neighbourhood—one at Antium and the other at Astura, a few miles further down the coast. It was at the former that he amused himself by "counting the waves." This favourite spot by the sea, although only recently brought into direct communication with Rome by means of a new line of railway, has already attracted considerable attention and promises to become popular with strangers, as a pleasant resort in the spring and early summer.

The climate is mild in winter and delightful during the months of April and May, while in summer and autumn it is said to be freer from malaria than the surrounding country. The position of the town is very fine, and nothing can surpass the beauty of the scenery as seen from the lighthouse. The picturesque little town of Nettuno, about a mile and a half distant, with the intervening woods of the Villa Borghese, form a pleasant feature in the landscape, and a more charming drive cannot be imagined than through these woods to Nettuno in the opening spring, when the trees are in full bud and the ground literally strewn with anemones and narcissus, while glimpses of the blue waters of the Tyrrhenian are obtained from several of the higher terraces above the villa. Good apartments are to be had, and the Hotel Milano, though small, is replete with every comfort.

The only spots which require notice in the Sabine and Tiburtine hills are Tivoli, Subiaco, and Olevano. The present route to Tivoli is across the Campagna by the steam tramway. About midway between

Rome and Tivoli, and a station of the tramway, are the famous baths of Albula. These waters, known to the ancient Romans as the Aquæ Albulæ, from their milky colour, contain very much the same mineral ingredients as those of Trajan's springs at Civita-Vecchia, and in addition, borax and a large quantity of sulphuretted hydrogen. So strongly does the sulphurous odour impregnate the air, that for a considerable distance before reaching the baths its presence can be detected. The waters are greatly resorted to by the Romans, and chiefly for affections of the skin.

The process of petrifaction of plants may be studied at these baths with comparative ease. All along the banks of the stream, reeds, grasses, carices and other plants may be found in every stage of incrustation, and beautiful specimens may be found in the neighbourhood. A short distance beyond the baths is Hadrian's Villa, and still further on, the tramway ascends through a lovely olive wood to the hill upon which Tivoli—the ancient Tibur—stands. No town in Italy occupies a more truly magnificent position, immediately overlooking, as it does, the valley of the Anio, with the splendid cascades formed by that stream.

In the early days of the Empire, Tivoli was the

favourite residence of many of the *literati* and statesmen of Rome, and the name "*superbum* Tibur," given to it by Virgil, though still remembered, is now only applicable to the beauty of its position and the surrounding hills, and it seems not unlikely that even this will be defaced if the scheme of its rulers is carried out, and the famous falls of the Anio are utilized for industrial purposes. Strangers rarely pass more than a few days at this lovely spot, and they merely visit it for the purpose of seeing the falls and making excursions in the neighbourhood. Probably many would make a longer sojourn if the hotels were more comfortable and more worthy of the place. Between twenty and thirty miles beyond Tivoli the town of Subiaco occupies a prominent position on a conical-shaped hill, partially surrounded by a double chain of mountains. The road from Tivoli follows, first the old Via Valeria, and afterwards the Via Sublacensis, constructed by Nero, and is one of remarkable beauty from the richness of the country through which it passes. This mountain town presents a striking contrast to that of Tivoli, for though the latter has in some respects a position superior to that of the former, yet Subiaco has less of the appearance of neglect and decay which so painfully impresses the visitor to Tivoli. The environs of the town are highly cultivated, and the gardens vie with each other in the richness of their produce and the loveliness of their flowers. Viewed from the Ponte S. Mauro at the head of the public walk, the position of the town is most advantageously seen.

Crowning the summit of the hill is the palace of the Abbot, which commands one of the finest and most extensive panoramas in Italy, while the two mountain chains which closely encircle the town readily account for its high temperature in the summer. It catches the first rays of the morning sun, and does not lose them till late in the afternoon, and although a considerable height above the sea and in the vicinity of high mountains, the heat in summer is very great. Interesting excursions can be taken in the neighbourhood, amongst them one to the Benedictine Monastery, which can only be reached by a bridle path leading from the left of the Ponte ; while to the right another path conducts to the site of the artificial lakes of Nero, in which that Emperor is said to have fished for trout with a golden net. Here he built a mountain villa which he called Sublaqueum—a name also applied to Subiaco. From Subiaco an excellent mountain road, constructed by Pius the Ninth, leads to Olevano, the favourite haunt of artists of every nationality. The road passes within a short distance of Civitella, the ancient Vitellia, perched on the summit of the beetling crags and so devoid of soil that the hardy mountaineers inhabiting it have been compelled to make a cemetery on a low adjacent spur, from which a magnificent view of the Campagna and the Hernician Mountains is obtained. A rapid descent soon brings the traveller to Olevano—the lovely spot which has so long exercised a fascination for artists. Any one who has stood on the verandah of the unpretending, homely, but comfortable Hotel Baldi, and seen the splendid panorama stretching towards Palestrina, will not be surprised that this picturesque little spot has tempted so many to delineate its features on canvas. The very name has a fragrance about it, and dates from mediæval times when the townsfolk had to pay a tax called Olibanum, for purchasing incense for the churches throughout the province.

The Alban towns are better known to strangers, being more easily reached than either Subiaco or Olevano, and are visited by them in large numbers towards the close of the Roman season. Frascati and Albano possess considerable advantages in the matter of accommodation, as well as many attractions both historic and archæological, and having what so few Italian resorts are able to boast of—

abundance of delightful shade in the woods and villa grounds of the neighbourhood, which are thrown freely open. They require very little to make them, what in fact they ought to be, pleasant and delightful summer retreats for those who do not wish to undergo the fatigue of railway journeys to more distant places.

The railway is now open direct to Frascati and Albano, and in a long summer day, travellers may leave Rome in the morning, taking the train to Frascati, a journey of less than an hour, and after a brief visit, proceed on donkeys to Tusculum, which is within easy walking distance of Frascati, and thence cross the beautiful valley lying between Tusculum and Montecavo, taking Rocca di Papa, and the so-called camp of Hannibal, on the way, and climbing to the summit of Montecavo by the lava-paved *Via Triumphalis*, a grassy platform is reached, crowned with a grand wych-elm, partially surrounded by some massive fragments of the ruins of the Temple of Jupiter Latiaris, which was destroyed towards the close of last century, for the purpose of building the Passionist Convent, which now occupies this incomparable site. From the rustic gate leading to one of the entrances of the convent, a panorama, which no words can adequately describe, spreads out before the traveller. Immediately beneath are the lovely lakes, Nemi and Albano, with the picturesque villages of the former, and Castle Gandolfo nestling at the head of the latter, while on a bold projecting spur, a few miles distant, is the picturesquely situated town of Civita Lavinia, surrounded by its vineyards, and so famous for its wine. It is more easy to descend the Via Triumphalis on foot than in the saddle, and the donkeys may be sent on before to wait at the bottom of the hill. On reaching Rocca di Papa the road to the left is taken, which conducts through charming forest glades to Nemi and Castle Gandolfo, and thence to Ariccia and Albano, from which the journey may be made back to Rome by rail in the evening. The hotels in Frascati and Albano are tolerably comfortable, and several excellent apartments are obtainable in both places. Rocca di Papa occupies a much higher altitude than either of these towns, being nearly 3,000 feet above the sea, and enjoys a fairly cool climate in summer, as well as freedom from malaria. My friend Dr. Steele, who spent several weeks in this neighbourhood a couple of summers ago, has furnished me with the following observations made by a friend :—

July.—Average mean temperature for month, 65° Fahr.

July.—Average difference between wet and dry bulbs, 5·4° Fahr.

August.—Average mean temperature for month, 63° Fahr.

August.—Average difference between wet and dry bulbs, 5·7° Fahr.

September.—Average mean temperature for month, 57° Fahr.

September.—Average difference between wet and dry bulbs, 3·8 Fahr.

There is no hotel at Rocca di Papa, but there are several comfortable dwelling-houses, and an enterprising, capable hotel-keeper might make a worse venture than to endeavour to make this beautifully situated mountain town attractive to foreigners. Its close proximity to the extensive grassy slope of Hannibal's camp—which, by-the-way, is said to have had nothing to do with Hannibal, but takes its name from the proprietors of the soil—and its nearness to Montecavo, and the delightfully green shady lanes of *La Fajola*, give it advantages possessed by no other town in the district; and with a good hotel and pension, in addition to the dwellings already to be had, Rocca di Papa should become one of the most popular and pleasant summer retreats near Rome. There are numerous other spots which might also be available if the communication between them and the capital was more direct; indeed, scattered all over this interesting, historic, and lovely district there are innumerable spots which, in the hands of a people like the Swiss, would have been ere now some of the most attractive inducements to visitors to prolong their stay in the City of the Seven Hills. Perugia and Siena, about midway between Rome and Florence, are favourably known to Italian travellers, and not a few of the visitors, both to Rome and Florence, spend the summer months in one or other of these towns, where the hotels are exceptionally good.

CHAPTER VIII.

Mineral Springs in Tuscany—Montecatini and Monsummano—La Spezia—Nervi—Tuscan Convents—Vallombrosa—Camaldoli and Sacro Eremo—Prato Vecchio—Alvernia—Bagni di Lucca—Mountains of Pistoia—Gavinana—San Marcello—Cutigliano—The Abetone——Forest of Abetone—Climate of Abetone—Certosa—Andorno.

THERE is no city in Italy so rich in summer quarters as Florence. In its immediate vicinity there are a great variety of pleasant spots, both at the seaside and among the mountains, and though several of these have only recently become known to strangers, they are already very popular, and the number of strangers who visit them is increasing every year.

The province of Tuscany, moreover, possesses mineral springs of great value, and from several of them the waters are sent to nearly all parts of the country. The waters of Montecatini are as well known in Rome and Naples as they are in Florence; and as a simple aperient, are equal to Friederichshall or Hunyadi Janos, while Castrocaro is richer in bromides and iodides than Kreuznach, and has a reputation in uterine affections in no way second to the famous German Spa.

The remarkable Grotto of Monsummano, about four miles from Montecatini, is favourably known—not only for the results obtained in chronic rheumatism, but cases of Eustachian deafness which appeared to defy all other treatment, received considerable benefit here. The Grotto is very dark, and as you enter nothing remarkable is felt in the way of temperature; but as you pass further in, it becomes hotter and hotter, and you are conscious of being in a great *Turkish* bath, and by the time you reach the *Inferno*, you are bathed in a profuse perspiration. One of the most intractable cases of throat deafness I ever knew, was completely cured by a few visits paid during two succeeding seasons to this hot air bath. The alkaline waters of Collalli, and the *earthy* waters of San Giuliano, Corsena, and Lucca, are also well known, the former in cases of gout and rheumatism, and the three latter in chronic cases with deposits in the joints, neuralgia, and some uterine disorders. The summer resorts in the neighbourhood of the Tuscan capital may be divided into three groups:—

Those at the seaside,
The Tuscan Convents now available for this purpose, and
The resorts in the Pistoia Mountains.

The seaside places within a short distance of Florence, and frequented by large numbers of Italians as well as foreigners, are Leghorn and the Ardenza, Via Reggio, and La Spezia. Leghorn is little more than two hours by rail from Florence, Via Reggio, a short distance further, on the railway to Genoa, while La Spezia is one hour beyond Via Reggio. At all three places there are most comfortable hotels, especially at Leghorn and Spezia, where they are as large and well appointed as any in the great Italian cities. At Via Reggio they are smaller, but not less comfortable, and what this favourite seaside resort lacks in the magnificence of its hotels, is more than compensated for by the extent and beauty of its sandy beach. The season begins about the middle of June, and continues till September, and both Spezia and Via Reggio have in recent years become favourably known as winter residences for invalids. In some respects Spezia is superior to Via Reggio as a winter resort, being more sheltered, and possessing numerous charming drives among the surrounding hills. As the hills overlooking the bay are all being fortified, the new military roads, now in course of construction in all directions, have opened up many lovely spots commanding magnificent views of the bay, while the scenery around Lerici is not surpassed by any upon the Cornice road. The Ligurian Riviera, extending from Spezia to Genoa, has been much frequented of late years, both in summer and winter; and Nervi, a few miles from Genoa, has acquired a great reputation in winter, although patients complain of the fewness of the walks in the neighbourhood. This Eastern Riviera has much to recommend it, both from the beauty of the views along the coast and the numerous sheltered nooks with which it abounds; and were the hotels as comfortable as they are on the Western Riviera, Sestri, Rapallo, Santa Margherita, and Nervi, would, ere long, be as popular as their rivals between Genoa and Cannes.

Several of the pleasantest summer quarters in the neighbourhood of Florence have long been known as the retreats of some of the monastic orders, and it is only within the past few years that they have become available as summer residences for strangers. All the Tuscan monasteries are delightfully situated, and several of them, having been suppressed by the Italian Government, are now opened as hotels or pensions. No more interesting and charming summer holiday could be taken than in visiting these ancient and instructive spots, all speaking of the grandeur of days gone by, and bearing silent testimony to the influence and devotion of men who have long since passed away, and which, though stripped of all that made them grand, yet retain the beauty of their situation and surroundings, of which no dynasty and no time can rob them. The traveller is completely awestruck with the traces of magnificence and ability which these ruined buildings present, and his wonder increases when he reflects upon the inaccessibility of their positions—even now some of them difficult to reach—positions, chosen for their retirement, safety, woods, pure air and water. Recently I visited three of these convents, and was favourably impressed with their suitability as summer quarters, and now at two of them there are most comfortable hotels, while at the third, any traveller is made welcome as the guest of the simple, unaffected, and genuinely kind *Frati*, and more clean cheerful rooms, with better fare, it would be difficult to find. These three monasteries form a group within the borders of Tuscany, and though some distance from each other, may, from the heights they occupy, be seen, the one from the other. They are also connected by good carriage roads, and mountain or bridle-paths, and can easily be visited by carriage, or across the mountains on foot. Starting from Florence, the traveller proceeds by rail to Pontassieve, a small station on the Roman railway, about half-an-hour from Florence, and near the foot of the mountain chain, on the slopes of which the Convent of Vallombrosa is situated. A pleasant drive of about two hours, passing Paterno and Tosi on the way, and the monastery is reached. From Vallombrosa there is a capital road, recently made, to Camaldoli, and thence to Alvernia. Two days would give ample time to visit all three. Travellers from Rome reverse this journey, and leave the railway at Arezzo, from whence a drive of about five hours brings them to Alvernia, and afterwards they proceed to Camaldoli and Vallombrosa by the route just described. Besides the carriage-road, there are several routes across the mountains by which the monasteries may be visted by the pedestrian. These mountain-paths lead through most beautiful scenery, and are much shorter than the retracing and windings of the public road. Moreover, they present no difficulties worth speaking of, and may be taken without a guide.

Vallombrosa is nearly 3,000 feet above the level

of the sea, and is situated in a beautifully shaded and sequestered spot among the vast pine forests. Like Certosa, its early history belongs to a very remote date. Although now suppressed, the convent buildings are all in the occupation of the Government as a school of forests. A large and commodious hotel has been erected within the past three years, and as the landlord is well acquainted with English ways, having lived for a lengthened period in English families, visitors may be assured of the comfort of the house. Vallombrosa is not shut in as Certosa is, and the splendid forests are sufficiently far removed to allow a free circulation of air. The climate is drier than the Val Pesio, and the water supply is abundant and delicious. The new road to the Consuma Pass is a pleasant drive, and the walks in the forests are endless, while the views from the lofty ridge of Pratomagno are exceedingly fine. Between 200 ft. and 300 ft. above the convent is the small cloister of *Il Paradisino*, perched upon a rocky cliff, and commanding a magnificent prospect of the surrounding mountains and valleys. This little *erie* is now a *dependence* of the hotel, and as the ascent from the valley below is somewhat steep, probably only *climbers* will be tempted to take up their abode in this veritable eagle's nest. The season lasts from May till October, but the hotel is open throughout the winter. The climate is delightful in early spring and autumn, and the temperature is similar to that of Abetone, though the rainfall is less. For the summer of 1881 I have a few observations of the weather, from which it appears that during July and August of that year rain fell in all eight times, and on three of these occasions it was only in light showers. The temperature during the same period was—

	July.	August.
In full sun, highest degree . .	89° Fahr.	90° Fahr.
In shade of forest, highest degree	74° ,,	75° ,,
In full sun, average degree . .	80° ,,	82° ,,
In shade, ,, ,, . .	68° ,,	68° ,,

Camaldoli and Sacro Eremo.—The famous Monastery of Camaldoli, with its dependent Monastery of Hermitages, lies in a small valley whose green slopes rise all around, giving it much more the appearance of an English than an Italian landscape. It is situated not far from the Casentino, or upper valley of the Arno, of which it commands a beautiful view. From Florence, the best starting point is the same as Vallombrosa. Leaving this little station the road towards the Consuma Pass rapidly ascends, having the famous Albizi Vineyards on the left, and Vallombrosa on the right. The Pass is about nine miles from Pontassieve, and is a bare, lonely, treeless height. We crossed it on a bright breezy summer day, but neither the sunshine nor the exhilarating air could divest us of a sense of the loneliness of this mountain brow. We had a pair of fine *iron grey* ponies, and drove along cheerily at a capital pace, and had not gone far down the gentle slope of the further side, when a gorgeous panorama burst upon our view. There lay spread out before us the rich fertile valley of the Casentino, so well known for its vineyards and thriving farms. Flowing down its stony bed, almost hid by overhanging vines, the Arno, here little more than a tiny mountain rivulet, appears like a silver thread running through the valley, a striking contrast to the muddy rapid river so familiar to visitors to Florence. Far away to the left, and nestling near the mountains, is the picturesque town of Stia, while immediately in front, Prato Vecchio lies, surrounded by vine slopes. Lower down the stream, Poppi and Bibbiena occupy commanding positions in the valley, and further away still the fertile Val di Chiana is seen stretching away towards Arezzo. Passing the ruined castle of Romena, we made a rapid descent, crossed the Arno by an old fashioned bridge, and put up at the quiet little inn of Prato Vecchio. After a couple of hours' rest we again set out, keeping the left bank of the Arno till Bibbiena was reached, when we left the main road and began the ascent to Camaldoli. At first the road led through a forest of oak and then chestnuts, and gradually as we reached higher ground the trees became smaller and less numerous, while the views of the surrounding country increased in extent and magnificence with each step of the ascent. At last we left all wood behind, and found ourselves slowly climbing another bleak and barren mountain ridge. The climb was long and slow, though the air was delightful. Having reached the summit, we caught the first glimpse of the deep dark forests around the convent, and were soon driving in the outskirts of the woods. By and by the bare mountain pass was soon forgotten as the well-kept avenues broke in upon our view, and we will not soon forget the peaceful homelike picture of the cows grazing contentedly on the grassy slopes, while the soft song of the haymakers floated gently towards us on this calm summer's eve. The convent is very large, and though suppressed, is still partly in the life occupation of the few monks who remain. The other portions are taken up by the forest department, and a very comfortable hotel under the charge of one of the best known Florentine hotel keepers. The buildings are situated at the bottom of the grassy hollow, and are hemmed in by mountain ridges which rise abruptly on all sides. The position, therefore, is not very favourable to a free and healthy circulation of air, and in midsummer the atmosphere is apt to be a little heavy and lifeless. Towards nightfall a copious dewfall begins, and continues throughout the night. The summer temperature is much the same as that of Certosa, although the altitude above the sea is nearly 2,000 ft. The walks in the immediate neighbourhood are very beautiful, and on the rising slopes and among the extensive forests, pleasant excursions, with little or no fatigue, can be taken. About a mile and a half above the convent, reached by a steep but good road, is the Hermitage or Sacro Eremo. The monastic regulations are much more severe here than at Camaldoli itself, and the whole plan of arrangement is different. There is not one large building for the monks as at the station below, but each monk has a small separate villa within its own little garden, very much in the same style as cottage hospitals are at present advocated. These monks live a very austere and solitary life, are only allowed to speak to each other three times a week, and to dine at the same table a dozen times in the course of the year; while every three hours both day and night, throughout the year, they assemble for worship in one or other of the chaste little chapels. Even in the depth of winter, when the snow lies deep on the ground, these self-imprisoned men leave their lonely, though comfortable little abodes to attend the required services of the Church during the silent hours of the night, and retire again without ever a friendly word being exchanged between them. The situation of this remarkable place is unrivalled by any of the other spots which we had visited. The chapels, villas, and gardens occupy a considerable plateau on the brow of a richly-wooded hill, from which the lovely parks and forests slope towards the larger valley below. Nothing could exceed the magnificence of the prospect from this enchanting spot, and no better sanatorium could be found throughout the whole of Italy. It is within immediate reach of the most perfect shade—it is not shut in by the mountains, and enjoys a freely-circulating, bracing and delicious air. The brotherhood is rapidly diminishing, and we venture to hope that ere long this delightful summer retreat will be as open to health seekers as the parent convent at the foot of the hill. The excursions in the neighbourhood are more interesting and of a grander description than those around any of the places previously described. One of the most beautiful is through the forest to the treeless summit of the *Prato al Soglio*, from whence a view of the Mediterranean and Adriatic is distinctly obtained, and further on by the same forest-path to the rocky fastnesses which give birth to the Arno and the Tiber.

Alvernia.—Sometimes also called La Verna, Monte Lerno, and Monte della Verna, is situated on the borders of Tuscany, and commands an extensive view of the Valley of the Arno and the hills beyond. Standing on the summit of the Prato al Soglio, behind Camaldoli, and looking towards Arezzo, a bold mountain-cone occupies the foreground of the landscape. It is partially surrounded by dark pine-forests, while in front and towards the Arno Valley it presents steep precipitous cliffs. On these cliffs the monastery is built. A good walker can easily go across the mountains from Camaldoli to La Verna in a summer afternoon; but to reach it by carriage the traveller must descend to the main road, to the point near Bibbiena where he left it on his way to Camaldoli. Having reached this point he again leaves the main road on the other side of

Bibbiena, and turns towards the great valley of the Corsalone. Another way is to walk to the little town of Soci, and begin the carriage journey there; but I think it is better to drive the whole distance in the way just described. From Bibbiena it takes between two and three hours to reach La Verna. It is a steep climb all the way, and the road leads through wild and uncultivated ground. At length a stony, undulating plain is reached, which is interspersed with marshy meadows. A small hamlet is now seen, and immediately above it rises the great sandstone mass of the Vernia—the highest point of which is about 4,000 ft. above the level of the sea. The buildings are very extensive, and are connected with the hamlet below by a steep paved way. The rock-hewn chambers under the monastery are memorable in connection with the history of St. Francis of Assisi. They are mainly situated on the verge of the precipice, and are reached by flights of stairs communicating by means of railed parapets. The views from these parapets are truly magnificent; while the gloomy cells and cloisters, so long the abode of St. Francis, give an interest to the place which none of the others possess. The monastery is not really suppressed, but is under the protection of the Municipality of Florence. This being the case it is as yet not available as a summer resort; which is the more to be regretted, as for position and purity of air it is equal to Abetone as a climate, and presents more attractions in the way of historic associations. The air is delightfully bracing, and the immense forests of beech and pine afford ample shade. It is to be hoped that ere long as much accommodation will be found here as at Camaldoli and Vallombrosa for summer visitors; meanwhile a number of rooms are maintained in the convent for the use of travellers, who must be gentlemen, and who are received as the guests of the monks. No charge is made and every comfort is amply provided. For the use of ladies, a small but commodious hospice is maintained at the little hamlet below, where they are received with the same liberality and on the same conditions as gentlemen are at the monastery itself.

The next group are all situated among the mountains of Pistoia, and are within easy reach of Florence. In this district, an altitude of from 3,000 feet to 4,000 feet will generally give a delightful summer climate, and there are numerous places at these heights along the whole range of the northern Apennines where seekers for health and recreation will find not only a pure and invigorating air, but also as charming a variety of scenery as in any country in Europe. Besides possessing a considerable number of pleasant mountain retreats, the district is also rich in mineral waters, among the best known being La Porretta, and the Bagni di Lucca, together with those mentioned at the beginning of this chapter.

La Porretta on the Pistoia and Bologna railway is situated at the mouth of one of the Gorges in the Apennines, and is nearly 1,200 feet above the sea. The waters are *saline*, of a high temperature, and several of the springs contain hydro-sulphuric acid. They enjoy a considerable reputation in cutaneous diseases. Season—June till September.

The baths of Lucca are the best known and most frequented of all the baths in Central Italy. They are situated in a beautiful valley about fifteen miles from the old town of Lucca, and until quite recently this was the only spot in Tuscany where foreigners ever thought of spending the summer. The baths themselves are unimportant, and are of the same *class* as those of San Giuliano. The "Bagni di Lucca" has been long better known as a favourite summer resort, and more prized for its *supposed coolness* than for its mineral waters. It has a great many advantages to recommend it. Here every comfort is to be found. The hotels and pensions are well kept, and the terms are very moderate, while the scenery in the neighbourhood is very beautiful; indeed there is everything fitted to make the place popular with visitors except *coolness*. The days are very hot, and not until the sun has well set, or in the early morning, can open-air life be enjoyed. The day is usually spent quietly indoors, or under the shade of some friendly tree, till the sun has lost his power.

Invalids and elderly people, who are incapable of much exertion, may pass a very comfortable summer at the Bagni di Lucca; but the healthy and strong, who are able for mountain work, would not be satisfied with the *climbing* around the Bagni, and even if they were, the great heat of the sun during the day would prevent the majority of visitors from attempting to take advantage of it. There is also a very heavy dewfall, an element in the climate which must be borne in mind in sending patients to this otherwise delightfully pleasant spot.

Further away towards the north, and nestling in the splendid pine-forests which skirt the highest carriage-way across the Apennines, are the now well known Abetone, Boscolungo, and Serrabassa; while lower down the valley stand Piano Sinatico, Cutigliano, San Marcello, and Gavinana, the former a shady little hamlet with its old-fashioned wayside inn, and the latter, three mountain village towns which are rapidly becoming popular as summer resorts. Before describing these spots separately, I propose to glance at the district generally, and the means of gaining access to it.

If the reader will look at a railway map, such as is found in any of the larger railway guide-books, he will find on the main line between Bologna and Turin the town of Modena, about an hour to the north of the former of these cities. Putting a pencil mark at Modena, let him now follow the line as far as Bologna and place another pencil mark there. Still tracing his way in the same manner, let him continue his journey as far as Pracchia, and thence to Pistoia—marking these towns as before. The district thus mapped will be found, roughly speaking, to form the two sides of a triangle, and the triangle will be completed if the reader will now draw a pencil line across the map from Modena to Pistoia. The portions of Modena and Tuscany thus inclosed contain all the summer quarters named above. The accessibility to this district will be readily understood when the reader is reminded that frequent trains go from Modena to Pistoia *viâ* Bologna, and *vice versâ*, every day, and that there is a magnificent carriage road from Modena to Pistoia, crossing the Apennines at Abetone, which in some parts is exceedingly beautiful; the whole distance being about ninety miles. There are several ways by which Gavinana, San Marcello, Cutigliano, and Abetone may be reached. First, the traveller coming from the north may quit the train at Modena and take a carriage there direct for Abetone. The distance is about sixty-two miles, and as a considerable portion of the road is an ascent he will be obliged to sleep at Pavullo, about twenty-five miles from Abetone. The drive from Pavullo to Abetone, by Barigazzo, Pieve à Pelago, and Fiumalbo, is both wild and beautiful. Another way, and a shorter, but quite as beautiful, is from Pracchia. The traveller proceeds by rail to Pracchia station, and here commences his carriage journey to Abetone. The drive takes about four and a half hours, and the road passes San Marcello and Cutigliano. Coming from Florence there are also two ways by which Abetone may be reached. The one is to go to Pracchia and take the journey just mentioned, or the traveller may leave the train at Pistoia and drive all the way to Abetone. The time occupied by this carriage journey is about eight hours, but it will well repay the lover of beautiful scenery who may choose to make it. Nothing, indeed, can be finer than the beauty of the views along the road. In four hours from Pistoia, San Marcello is reached, and here a halt is usually made to take refreshment and feed the horses. Making a fresh start, Abetone can easily be reached in another four hours. Carriages can always be had at Modena and Pistoia; but travellers quitting the train at Pracchia would do well to send to San Marcello for conveyances to come and meet them, as they are not always to be had at the station. The road from Pracchia goes along the left bank of the Reno for nearly three miles, and joins the Pistoia-Modenese road, about seven miles from San Marcello. Less than an hour's drive after leaving Pracchia brings the traveller to the top of a rather steep ascent, from which he can see San Marcello, charmingly situated in the valley below. At Oppio, a rugged-looking hill-road turns off abruptly to the right, and after winding for two or three miles, first through roughly-cultivated ground, and afterwards through very fine chestnut woods, reaches Gavinana.

Gavinana.—Leaving the main Pistoia-Modenese road at Oppio, the traveller ascends by a good and recently-made road, which at first leads through patches of cultivated ground, but soon enters the chestnut forest. The trees in this forest are very old, and many of them have a peculiarly gnarled and fantastic appearance. Nothing is seen of the village, which nestles among the rich green foliage, until the traveller is close upon it. We drove into it on a bright pleasant day in the end of June, and were struck with the beauty of the village surroundings. We had a glimpse of it from the main road two years before, and thought that nothing could exceed the loveliness and picturesqueness of its position. Leaving the village, we turned our steps towards the grand old forest, and were particularly charmed with the fine park which lies between the houses and the mountains: everywhere a carpet of the richest green met the eye, with here and there scattered up and down its lovely glades clumps of fine old trees which afforded much more efficient shade than is usually found in chestnut woods. Gavinana is situated on an eminence on the southern slope of the Apennines under Monte Crocicchio, and is about 2,500 feet above the level of the sea. It may be described as a small mountain village town in which several good houses could be found suitable for summer quarters. It has a supply of excellent water, the air is moderately dry and unstimulating, and from its proximity to the chestnut-forest has an abundance of shade. It presents, therefore, many elements which, if developed, are capable of making it a most desirable summer residence. There is an excellent hotel (Ferruccio) kept by Signor and Mrs. Cerimboli. It is only a few years since the hotel was opened, and it is already known as one of the best in the district. Under the management of its present enterprising proprietor, who is sparing no expense in carrying out improvements to render his hotel a comfortable residence, Gavinana will become one of the most pleasant spots as a summer resort for families.

From Gavinana, San Marcello is reached by a rough but good walking road. This is a favourite walk with the visitors at Gavinana: the distance between the two places is little more than a mile and a half.

San Marcello is about 2,100 feet above sea-level, and until quite recently has been the most frequented spot in summer among the Pistoia Apennines, chiefly because it is easy of access, being situated on the main road, and possessing advantages which the other places had not, in the shape of comfortable houses, hotels, post and telegraph offices, &c. It is, however, inferior in point of climate to either Gavinana or Cutigliano, being several hundred feet lower than both these places, and, what is of more consequence, much worse off in respect of shade. During the summer months the place is completely enveloped in dust, and there is no shade worthy of the name within a considerable distance of the town. The absence of shade is perhaps the greatest defect of San Marcello as a summer quarter. There is also a heavy dewfall. However, the air is pure and the nights delightfully cool, but the visitor would be compelled to spend the greater part of the day within doors. It is indeed impossible to be much in the open air except in the evening or early morning, and invalids and others who expect to find shady and pleasant walks in the woods would be greatly disappointed in San Marcello—and to some extent, although to a less degree, the same remark is applicable to Cutigliano. To those, however, who would be content to spend their day indoors and enjoy a pleasantly cool morning or evening stroll, San Marcello has several advantages. There is at least one fairly well-kept hotel and one good café, about which there is always more or less life during the summer evenings. Being moreover a good-sized village town, there is not the same isolation felt which some might complain of in higher mountain places. About midway between Gavinana and

San Marcello Madame Piccioli of Florence has opened a summer *pension*. The house is very large and commodious, and situated in its own grounds at some distance from the main road and close to a chestnut wood. Two small mountain streams which pass near the house are to be utilized for a bathing establishment. The position I consider superior to San Marcello, but not equal to Gavinana. However, what the *pension* may lack in position it has more than made up for by the internal arrangements. The house is replete with every comfort, and the grounds around it begin already to have a very home-like appearance. Beautiful flower-beds surround the building, and a well-kept prato (lawn) stretches away towards the wood, while here and there small rustic bridges are thrown across the streams, which give the place the air of a comfortable residence.

Cutigliano is about six miles higher up the valley than San Marcello. It is, according to Professor Tigri, about 2,200 feet above the level of the sea, and has a commanding position at a considerable elevation above the Lima and on the left bank of that stream. It is fully a mile from the main road. The Lima is crossed by a substantial bridge, and then a very steep but well made zigzag road leads up to the little town. During the past few years Cutigliano has been an important summer place, and now numbers amongst its other advantages a club, café, post and telegraph offices. The situation of the town is very fine. It stands boldly out on the steep hill-side which forms the north bank of the Lima, and commands a magnificent view of the far-reaching chestnut forests which fill the valley of that river. Beyond these forests the first glimpse of the mountains around Abetone is obtained—the two peaks of the Libro Aperto (open book) conspicuously occupying the foreground, while the splendid valley of the Sestaione is seen extending far away towards the higher peak of the Tre Potenze. Cutigliano being on the very edge of, or rather encircled by the chestnut forests, has much more to offer in the way of rambles through the woods than San Marcello, but even here it is necessary to spend the hottest hours of the day in the house, especially on the part of those who are unable to make excursions among the higher mountains and to bear the heat of the sun and the fatigue which they entail. Pleasant bits of shade are found here and there in the woods, which enable visitors to sit out of doors during the greater part of the day, excepting the midday hours, when the sun is powerful. The climate of Cutigliano is cool and pleasant.

There is one fair hotel and three good *pensions*, two of them being English. Madame Rochat is well known to visitors to Florence, and Mrs. Jennings, who is now in her excellent new house—La Villa— offers every comfort to English families.

Just above Cutigliano, but on the Abetone road, and close to the Ponte Sestaione, a very good hotel has been recently opened by the proprietor of the Hotel Milano in Florence: two miles higher up is Piano Sinatico, with its rather comfortless inn, and a mile beyond is Piano Cici, which some day may become a pleasant summer quarter. Still further on towards Abetone is Cechetto, situated at the lower edge of the pine forests, where a comfortable villa may sometimes be obtained.

THE ABETONE.—This delightful retreat presents a striking contrast to the places which have been already briefly described, and in fact so great is the contrast that they cannot well be compared together. The great desideratum at Gavinana, San Marcello, and Cutigliano was *shade* in addition to a sufficiently cool atmosphere. At Abetone *shade* can be had in perfection and in abundance. Indeed the *life* at Abetone is very much what it would be among the higher altitudes in Switzerland, or in the north of Scotland. The flora of the valleys and sub-alpine regions is almost identical with that of the north of Scotland, and the temperature during the whole of the summer, from the 1st of July till the end of September, is that of an ordinary English summer. During my stay of nearly three months I made careful observations of the climate, the results of which, together with those of the following summer, made with better instruments, are given below.

Abetone has two names—Boscolungo and Abetone; the former given in reference to the extent of the pine forests, and the latter from the fact of an immense silver fir having been felled during the construction of the road from Modena to Pistoia. The Italian name for a pine-tree is *Abete*, and for a great pine-tree *Abetone*.

The forests are composed almost entirely of pines, of which there are several varieties. The spruce and the silver fir are the most abundant; next comes the larch; and lastly, here and there in the depth of the forest are to be found solitary specimens of the hardy Scotch fir.

Leaving San Marcello, the road rapidly descends till it reaches the turbulent Lima, which at this spot is crossed by means of an ancient *turreted* bridge. Immediately after crossing this bridge the road divides—the one to the right going to Abetone, the other to the left to the Bagni di Lucca. From this point to the Bagni di Lucca is about ten miles, the road passing through some of the finest scenery of the lower Lima. Taking the right-hand road we at once turn towards Abetone. An easy ascent soon brings us in sight of Cutigliano, looking from her commanding position like the queen of the valley. Shortly after passing Cutigliano the massive Ponte Sestaione is crossed and the real ascent to Abetone begins. The road now winds through the great chestnut forest. Slowly climbing up, first leading to the right, then towards the left, and again turning back upon itself, till by a series of the most picturesque windings the chestnut forest is cleared and the zone of beech is reached a little way above Piano Cici. This magnificent mountain road, built in some places of solid masonry, and enlivened at several of its most beautiful *turns* by quaint-looking little hamlets, is a standing memorial of the splendid engineering abilities of the famous monk, Leonardo Ximenes. The upper valley of the Lima is much wilder than the lower, and the stream pours over its rocky bed in a ravine of immense depth. The road climbs along the south side of this gorge, and the traveller is reminded that he has left the chestnut forest behind, not only by the presence of beech-trees everywhere around him, but by the freshness and strength of the air. Invariably at this part of the road he quits his carriage and pushes on ahead enjoying the delicious cool breeze, after the great heat which he had experienced only a couple of miles below. For nearly three miles nothing is seen but beech on the mountain-sides, till at length just below Cechetto a small belt of larch is reached, on the right side of the road. At this point the long line of forests first becomes visible, and away in the distance rising up between the traveller and the western sky is a conspicuous wooded hill crowned with stately beeches of great age. This hill marks the summit of the *pass*, which is now scarcely three miles off. The road here is comparatively level, and for some distance skirts the edge of the great forest which forms one of the watersheds of the finest of all the streams of the higher Apennines—the Sestaione. Far down in the depths away towards the right, the Lima, here little more than a tiny rill, speeds its way along its almost unseen bed, while rising up on the steep hill-sides beyond, the picturesquely situated little hamlets of Rivoreta, Melo and Bicchiere are seen. Higher up, the valley becomes narrower, and the magnificent spruce and silver pines line the road on both sides. About half a mile from the summit there is a break in the forest, and between the road and one of the sources of the Lima lies the nursery ground of the Forest Department, while almost opposite is the handsome residence of the officer in charge of the forests and the recently built Albergo della Lima. Immediately adjoining the nursery ground is a beautiful and extensive undulating park—the general rendezvous of those of the visitors who limit their excursions to the neighbourhood of the hotel. On the upper edge of this park the Hotel Orsatti is situated, commanding a most lovely view of the valley below, of the Cappel d'Orlando, and away beyond, of the Apennine range towards the Corno alle Scale and the Lago Scaffaiolo. Beside the hotel are the parish church and the post-office. Just above the church is another park, commanding a still more splendid view than the one below, and which is the spot of all others likely to become ere long the site of an important summer sanatorium. After passing the upper park the road again enters the forest at one of its most beautiful turns, and a walk of three minutes brings the traveller to the summit of the pass—which is the frontier of the two old duchies of Tuscany and Modena.

Emerging from the deep shade of the lovely forest-road, the traveller sees before him two simple but picturesque stone pyramids which mark the boundary between the two provinces; but he is unprepared for the splendid panorama which bursts upon his view the moment his feet touch the boundary line. Suddenly he finds himself at the head of a magnificent valley which stretches away before him as far as the eye can reach. The valley is bounded on the left by the forests and alps of Faidelo, and on the right by the Apennine chain, with Cimone lifting its hoary head against the bluest of blue skies.

Immediately in front, Monte Modino, a bold, rugged mountain ridge, abruptly crosses and partly breaks up the valley; and away beyond it, rising up range after range, the vast mountain chains of the Neggio and Modena alps are distinctly seen. At the head of the valley and close to the pyramids, and in full view of this beautiful landscape, stands the *pension* of Serrabassa, kept by Dr. Major.

One feature of importance in the climate of Abetone is, that the range between day and night is less than in some mountain resorts. In some Swiss places a difference of 30° to 40° Fahr. between the day and night temperatures is not a very unusual experience, and in regard to *dryness* of air, the relative humidity may be about 80 or 90 per cent. during the morning and evening, and as low as 35 or even 30 after mid-day. Exposure to these extremes of cold and dampness, either in the open air or through windows opened for the purposes of ventilation, entails considerable risk, and is the great source of inflammatory affections of the throat and air passages during the summer months. For the delicate as well as for the healthy, the relation between the day and night temperature should be such as will admit of free ventilation during the entire twenty-four hours. At Abetone the day temperature during summer varies from 60° to 72° Fahr., and the night temperature from 45° to 55° Fahr. All through my stay of two summers the windows of my bedroom were always more or less open day and night. The following observations made during this period show that the dangers which are incidental to many mountain resorts north of the Alps are experienced in a very much less degree at Abetone.

	July, 1879.	July, 1880.
In full sun, max. temp.	89° Fahr.	94° Fahr.
Average for month	82° ,,	86° ,,
In shade of forest, max.	67° ,,	73° ,,
Average for month	62° ,,	66° ,,
In sitting-room (E) max.	65° ,,	68° ,,
Average for month	61° ,,	64° ,,
Greatest cold *outside* during night	44° ,,	47° ,,
Average for month	49° ,,	52° ,,
Black bulb *in vacuo*, max.	108° ,,	111° ,,
Average for month	$105\frac{1}{2}$° ,,	107° ,,
Wet and dry bulb, max. diff.	8° ,,	9° ,,
Average during month	$5\frac{1}{2}$° ,,	$6\frac{3}{4}$° ,,

The month of July in 1879 set in with a few stormy days, during which rain fell heavily. Rain fell in all seven times during the month, but on no occasion was it so continuous as to leave less than two or three hours every day for open-air exercise.

July of 1880 was warmer than the preceding year, and rain fell only *twice* during the entire month.

	Aug., 1879.	Aug., 1880.
In full sun, max. temp.	91° Fahr.	94° Fahr.
Average for month	84° ,,	87° ,,
In shade of forest	69° ,,	75° ,,
Average for month	64° ,,	67° ,,
In sitting-room, max.	68° ,,	73° ,,
Average for month	63° ,,	66° ,,
Greatest cold *outside* during night	46° ,,	48° ,,
Average for month	51° ,,	55° ,,
Black bulb *in vacuo*, max.	110° ,,	112° ,,
Average for month	106° ,,	108° ,,
Wet and dry bulb, max. diff.	8° ,,	10° ,,
Average for month	6° ,,	7½° ,,

The whole of August, 1879, was exceptionally fine. Rain fell *four* times during the month, but the amount that fell was small. During several days the mid-day sun was hot, and *on one occasion* the thermometer did not fall below 60° during the night. In 1880 the weather was very beautiful till the 20th of the month, when it became showery, and then rain fell, more or less, every day till the end of the month.

	Sept., 1879.	Sept., 1880.
In full sun, max. temp.	85° Fahr.	
Average for month	78° ,,	
In shade of forest	63° ,,	
Average for month	59° ,,	*No record for September.*
In sitting-room	62° ,,	
Average for month	57° ,,	
Greatest cold *outside* during night	36° ,,	
Average for month	45° ,,	
Black bulb *in vacuo*, max. diff.	98° ,,	
Average for month	92° ,,	
Wet and dry bulb, max. diff.	6½° ,,	
Average for month	5° ,,	

September began with a slight thunderstorm, after which for a few days the weather was beautifully fine. On the 6th there was a second thunderstorm, which was followed by a fortnight of the most splendid weather. Rain fell twelve times during the month, but, as in July and August, it rarely was so continuous as to prevent visitors from enjoying a part of their accustomed open-air life.

Abetone is about 4,500 feet above the level of the sea, and is situated at the head of a beautiful wide and well-wooded valley which runs in a south-westerly direction towards the lower Lima. The valley is bounded on the north and east by the Apennine range, while the extensive forests, lying between the Lima and the Sestaione, form its western side. Although in the neighbourhood of mountains of considerable height, they are sufficiently far away to secure a thoroughly free circulation of air. It is in no sense a valley shut in by mountains. The summit of the pass which forms the head of the valley is the highest carriage-way across the northern Apennines.

The climate is very dry and the temperature moderate. The days are not too hot and the nights are not too cold. Open-air life may be enjoyed here as freely as in England, and under a brighter and bluer sky. For invalids the comparative evenness of temperature is an important element, as it enables them to be much in the open air and to have the benefit of free ventilation during the night, without the risks which are so frequently encountered in high mountain resorts. I have visited almost every well-known spot likely to furnish a summer quarter in Central and North Italy, but nowhere did I find a climate superior to that of Abetone, or a place surrounded by more beautiful scenery. Besides the matter of climate, there are other considerations which give value to Abetone as a summer residence—

It is of easy access from any part of Italy.

It affords abundance of the most perfect shade, and the number of walks in the pine-forests is endless.

The roads are all kept in excellent order, and pleasant drives can be taken to Cecchetto on the one side, and to Fiumalbo and Pieve à Pelago on the other side of the pass.

The mountain excursions in the neighbourhood are very fine, and there is an unlimited supply of delicious ice-cold water. Comfortable accommodation can now also be secured. There are several *Contadini* houses, small, but pleasant and cheerful-looking, which visitors can rent for themselves. The handsome large villa built by my friend Professor Gardini is now finished, and is a *dependence* of the Hotel Orsatti. There is also an excellent *pension*, kept by Dr. Major, where every comfort can be had, and two hotels—Ferrari and Orsatti. The hotel Ferrari is a new house and is well spoken of. Hotel Orsatti has been established for many years. The house is beautifully situated, and the landlady is English.

In addition to these there are several very pleasant summer spots in Piedmont, of which I will only refer to the two following :—

Certosa di Pesio.—This monastery is picturesquely situated in the upper valley of the Pesio, a wild mountain torrent which flows close to the convent buildings. It is about 3,000 feet above the level of the sea, and is within easy reach, either by way of Turin or Savona. Travellers from the north coming by Mont Cenis break their journey at Turin; thence take rail to Cuneo, a quaint, thriving old town, about three hours' journey from Turin. Here a comfortable halt can be made at the *Barro di Ferro*, from whence a diligence starts twice a day for Certosa. Cuneo is the centre of several diligence routes, amongst others, one to Nice, across the maritime alps, by the Col di Tenda. Another way of reaching Certosa is by Savona, a station on the railway between Nice and Genoa. From Savona there is a short branch line to Mondovi, and from Mondovi the remainder of the journey is made by carriage. The distance from Mondovi to Certosa is about four hours, the same as from Cuneo. The two roads join at Chiusa di Pesio. Being anxious to have a good look of the country, which was quite new to me, I started from Cuneo at two o'clock, about four hours before the ordinary time of starting for the diligence. The first part of the journey lay through a flat but very fertile plain. The day was hot, and the road very dusty, and the drive at that hour—the hottest in all the day—would have been anything but agreeable but for the rivulets of clear water, which, flowing rapidly along both sides of the road, were freely used for irrigating the fields, giving them a delightfully fresh appearance. After a drive of less than two hours we entered the Val Pesio, and enjoyed the ample shade afforded by the walnut and chestnut trees overhanging the road which follows the right bank of the stream. In some places the lower valley ranges from half a mile to a mile in breadth, and is everywhere highly cultivated—the grain fields being watered by small channels led from the bright, clear torrent. Gradually ascending the beautiful valley—dotted here and there with clean, thriving-looking hamlets—the steep mountain ridges draw closer together until it seems as if the road must end in a rocky *cul de sac.* Climbing still higher, the valley becomes narrower, till there appears only room for the river and the road. The snowy mountain ridge crossing the head of the valley now comes distinctly into view; and with it the first glimpse of the convent, beautifully situated on the other side of the stream. Leaving the road, we enter a shady path of stately elms, and cross the Pesio by means of an ancient covered bridge. A few steps more and we are within the enclosure formed by the magnificent old building. After a bath and a comfortable dinner I sauntered forth to view the surroundings of my new abode and enjoy the cool evening air. The buildings form a splendid pile, and are bounded on three sides by a large corridor or covered verandah; the rooms are tastefully furnished with every convenience, and are scrupulously clean. Yet, notwithstanding, I confess to a feeling of regret at seeing the grand old building converted into a modern *pension*. The grounds are no longer kept in first-rate order; but still they are beautiful. Fine old terraced walks, covered with rich greensward, extend up into the woods to a considerable distance, and in the vicinity of the house there are a number of rare flowering-trees and shrubs. The walks in the neighbourhood are numerous, shady, and beautiful, and the view towards the head of the valley from the old bridge cannot be surpassed. The clear crystal waters of the Pesio not only add to the beauty of the landscape, but are a source of great enjoyment to the disciples of old Izaak Walton. The earliest records of this interesting place date as far back as 1200, and in recent times it has passed through several hands. When Napoleon annexed Piedmont in the early part of this century he suppressed the convent, and it afterwards became a somewhat famous bathing establishment, to which large numbers of the nobility resorted. It is now inferior to its neighbour and rival, Valdieri, as a *stabilmento dei*

Bagni, and for many years past has been much less known than formerly, especially to strangers; but again it is attracting considerable attention, and Mons. Cherbasse, from Nice, who directs the summer pension, is anxious to make it as comfortable and complete as possible, and in this he has succeeded. The best months to visit Certosa are July and August. The position of the convent is very much shut in, being almost entirely surrounded by high mountain ridges, and in consequence, the climate is apt to be rather damp in June and cold in September. In July and August, when the weather is sunny, the climate is very fine. The days are never oppressively warm, and the nights are pleasantly cool. The average temperature during these months, indoors, is 60° Fahr. about mid-day, and 50° to 56° in the night. Within the immediate precincts of the house there is ample shade, so that invalids and children can spend much of their time in the open air.

Andorno. Half an hour's drive from the station of Biella, about midway between Turin and Milan, is the beautifully situated village of Andorno, at the entrance of the valley of the Cervo. The weather becomes hot in August, but for the early summer and autumn it is one of the most delightful spots in

S

North Italy. The hotel is not surpassed for excellence by any with which I am acquainted, and Signor Sella, the proprietor, spares no pains to make his visitors comfortable. The walks in the neighbourhood are very fine, and some magnificent snowy peaks overlook the valley beyond, in which are situated the well-known Stabilmenti dei Bagni of the two *Sanctuarii*.

Adjoining the grounds of the hotel is a large, comfortably appointed hydropathic establishment, where the most recent appliances in *hydropathy* are to be found. The various forms of electric baths are especially well arranged, and many important cases were under treatment upon the occasion of my visit.

CHAPTER IX.

Influence of the Mediterranean—Effects of Italian Climate upon Chronic Disease—Earliest Symptoms of Broken Health—Importance of these Early Symptoms—Description of Early Symptoms—More Advanced Symptoms—Personal Experiences—Cases Suitable for Rome—Holiday for Professional Men—Cases Unsuitable for Rome—Abuse of Quinine.

THE classes of invalids to whom an Italian atmosphere is likely to prove curative, include those forms of disease which require a frequent removal to receive the full benefit to be derived from change of air, and therefore the consideration of the kind of patients for whom Rome might prove a desirable winter residence involves some knowledge of other parts of Italy where the climate would be auxiliary to that of Rome. There is, as stated in a previous chapter, certain climatal conditions which may be said to belong to Italy generally; but in many other respects there is a very great difference between the resorts on the eastern and those on the western coast, and this is due, not so much to latitude as to the presence of great mountain chains, which, while they afford complete protection to the one half of the Peninsula, leave the other half, exposed. The Alps and the Apennines form together a great protecting screen to the north-east, as will be readily seen by consulting a map of Northern Italy with the adjacent countries of France and Switzerland. The great Swiss alpine chain terminates somewhat sharply in the plains of Piedmont, in the well-known passes of Mont Cenis, the St. Bernard, and the Simplon, and is continued towards the Mediterranean, where, at Nice, it takes the name of the Maritime Alps. From this point the mountains skirt the shore of the Gulf of Genoa, taking at first a north-easterly direction, and afterwards south-easterly as far as Lucca. Beyond Genoa the Alps merge into the Apennines, and, leaving the coast, they occupy the centre of the Peninsula as far south as Reggio. Italy is therefore divided into two sections by these mountain chains, and the climate of the eastern section is colder than that of the western. The mountains vary in height from four to ten thousand feet, and constitute a barrier which protects the whole of the western coast from the north-east winds of Central and Northern Europe, while the eastern, or Adriatic coast-line, from being exposed to these winds, is much colder in winter and spring. Another important feature in the climate of the western coast is its exposure to the warm south-west winds and warm Mediterranean currents, which impart a mildness to it peculiar to itself. Invalids who may therefore desire to pass the winter and spring in Italy, have a choice of sheltered nooks along the western coast, in any one of which they might comfortably locate themselves. To many, these spots might be convenient halting places on their way to Rome, as Perugia, Siena, Florence, and Venice are on their homeward journey.

In a previous chapter, when discussing the prevalent diseases and mortality in Italy and in England, it was found that the death-rate in the former was not only higher than in the latter, but that it was due to diseases of an opposite character to those which cause the largest proportion of deaths in England. That, in fact, while chronic disease predominated in England, the reverse was true of Italy, and this experience was so general throughout the whole country, affecting all classes of the community, as to leave no doubt that climate was an essential factor in the production of these results. A study of the main features of the Italian climate already described will readily show sufficient ground for this conclusion. The dryness of the air, without excessive heat or cold, rendering it unnecessary for the mucous membranes to put on their slimy coats of mucus, they are in a more active condition for the work of absorbing oxygen, digesting, extracting nourishment or water, or whatever else they require to do. They are filled with blood, and pass it on rapidly with its fresh burden of new life to the tissues.

The comparative warmth of the air, the shortness of the winter, and the abundance of sunshine, render it possible for all—invalids included—to be a good deal in the open air, and that the sunlight is a great reddener of the blood no one now disputes. While the wakefulness and activity of the nervous system renders the use of alcohol less necessary, and thus prevents that torpidity of the vital processes and degeneration of tissue so commonly seen in the chronic illnesses of northern climates, and which prove so fatal to many invalids; moreover, by the diet containing animal food less rich in fat, is avoided the rancidity so familiar to us in slow digestion which renders it innutritious, and which we have therefore to counteract by our remedies. The improved digestion implied in the removal of rancidity must be an important element in the supply of new material to the worn out tissues to replace the degenerated and the degenerating. These effects, if they have been traced to their true source, are convincing evidence of the value of the Italian climate in those cases of chronic diseases accompanied by degeneration of tissue, and in which the vital processes require hastening, and we may expect from it increased activity in the repair of tissues, increased activity of circulation to supply the material of repair, and of nervous energy to regulate the whole. In short, we may hope for a renewal of life, the converse and the cure of that half death which so many experience who are victims to some chronic wasting malady.

The pathological conditions which underlie these chronic degenerating processes, appear to be due to a weakness of blood circulation, which is the common link uniting them all; whereas the acute affections, which are characteristic of Italian medical practice, are marked by activity of circulation and a high degree of arterialization of the blood. Thus the diseases of the two countries are the opposites of one another, and clinical experience has shown that the climate of Italy has a powerfully *renewing* influence in the case of those convalescents who do not continue to convalesce, whose convalescence is impeded, and who are in danger from the kindred conditions of general atrophy and of deficient regenerative power, which are apt to appear in the course of so many chronic illnesses. These are just the cases in which medicines are so often powerless to arrest the progress of the degenerating process in which the clear, dry, sunny air of Italy is so potent to renew to more vigorous life those morbid states of constitution which, if left to themselves, pursue their slow but steady march to the grave. It is not, therefore, any particular spot in Italy the air of which alone is endued with these *quickening* powers; the *main* climatal conditions are found to be much the same throughout the Peninsula, except in the matter of temperature in winter, when the section lying to the east of the mountain chain is decidedly colder than the west, although in summer not much difference is observable between the two. There is, however, in winter, abundance of sunshine on the eastern side, as well as on the western, and for a certain class of invalids who require frequent change and a crisp, bracing air, many of the places on the Adriatic coast afford a delightful climate for a winter sojourn. In enumerating the classes of patients who are likely to reap benefit from a residence in the Italian capital, I will arrange them in the order of the seasons, the winter in Rome being marked by the highest mortality, the spring next, then the autumn, and the summer least of all. There is a large and increasing class of invalids who are not the subjects of any *known* disease—that is, an examination of all their organs would reveal no organic change in any of them, and, yet though no part could be pointed out as *diseased*, the patient might be weak and ill—indeed, very ill—and what the cold science of the physician could not detect, is often apprehended in a shrewder manner by the observation of those near and dear to the patient, who see a change which the physician fails to observe, and to whose loving eyes matters appear far from well, while as yet no change has taken place in any viscus to a degree capable of being detected by the attendant, and of being called by a specific name. Sometimes this weakness is induced, as, for example, by long-continued sedentary occupations, when the contractile fibres of the heart and arteries become sluggish from want of use; or, again, by anxiety of mind, when the nervous energy is withdrawn from the involuntary muscles, or by exhausting debaucheries. In other cases it is brought on by the combined influence of physical fatigue and anxiety, as in the prolonged nursing of a relative; sometimes it is congenital; sometimes it is hereditary; and it may originate in a single organ, though more frequently it begins by affecting the whole constitution, and only after a period of silent progress does it manifest itself in a diseased heart or kidneys, in a softened brain, or a paralytic seizure. Long before these results are reached, however, and before suspicions are aroused in the mind of the physician, the relatives and friends may be able to satisfy themselves that all is not right, and they speak of broken health, or a threatening break-up.

The following incident—the earliest lesson I received in practical medicine—produced a lasting impression upon my mind. Mr. B., aged fifty, a successful merchant who had amassed a large fortune, began to manifest symptoms of irritability and sleeplessness, and complained frequently of uneasy sensations in his head. It was during a great commercial crisis, and though his personal affairs were untouched, he shared with others the anxiety of the time, and devoted himself a little more closely to business matters; but, beyond this, there was no apparent cause for the *change* which had come over him. His wife became anxious at times, when she saw him so unlike himself, and so fitful about his food. Some days he would eat as usual, on other days he would take nothing. At last she persuaded him to consult

IMPORTANCE OF THESE EARLY SYMPTOMS.

the family physician, which he did the same day, and, on his return home in the evening, in answer to a question as to what Dr. D.'s opinion was, he replied, "He says I am all right, and only want a bottle of champagne for my dinner; but I am afraid he scarcely knows how ill I feel." Next morning he was found dead, having died by his own hand. Probably had more thoughtful interest been taken in this case, instead of pooh-poohing it, and a change of air and scene been recommended, it might have saved a valuable life. It is important to recognize as a definite disease, this period of *broken health*, which so often shows itself before the various degenerations referred to manifest themselves, and to know that however much their final symptoms may differ, their origin, and the mode of curing them, when it is not too late, are similar. Dr. King Chambers, himself a patient sufferer from one of the forms of retarded convalescence alluded to, describes the condition in a classic manner. He says:—

"The approaches of the enemy are very insidious. The sufferer is unable to draw any clear picture of the symptoms; no one place is painful, and no one function of life absolutely abnormal; yet he feels himself less capable than formerly of transacting the ordinary work of life; the business letter, that it was lately a pleasure to write, first loses its interest, and then becomes a burden; the worries of the kennel and of the parish, of the patients, or the clients, become so intolerable that he gives up his very hobbies. Then he grows stiff, and knocked up after the daily shorter constitutional; going up hill is especially fatiguing, though he does not suffer from shortness of breath. The night's rest is almost always insufficient. The patient drops asleep in getting into bed out of utter weariness, but soon wakes up again, and is restless for the remainder of the time spent in bed. The ears buzz, and the back of the neck aches, and the bowels keep up a fidgetty grumble, and nothing more. Then he feels uncomfortable after a moderate meal; his meat oppresses him, and his wine flushes him. As time goes on, he finds he can take less and less alcohol with advantage to himself; he says 'he feels to want it,' but that it does not do him good as in days gone by. Symptoms of defective circulation are seldom absent; the knees and ankles are stiff and swelled of an evening, and as he stands about at his morning wash, he sees his feet flushed and congested with stagnant blood. Mysterious pains in the back and side are felt after sitting down or riding for even short periods; often a dull discomfort at the back of the neck seems as it were going to be a sick headache, but does not prove so. The urine is usually pale; it irritates the bladder, especially in the forenoon, and causes frequent micturition. There is often flatulence after exertion of mind or body and apparently independent of the quantity of food taken.

Perhaps at first all this is attributed to what is called 'derangement of stomach;' but observation of the action of the bowels shows not enough to account for the continued ill health. The stools are, indeed, scanty and softer than natural; but they occur at the usual hours daily, and are rarely diarrhœic. The wind from the intestines, when flatulence is present, seldom has that fœtor of sulphuretted hydrogen so characteristic of dyspeptic decomposition. That is to say, it has not naturally; but if purgatives are taken, then the indigestion, which I have described as absent, is sometimes artificially induced. Soon the complexion loses its transparency, and acquires a faded dingy or grey hue; though, if there is any fixed colour in the skin, this becomes darker and more fixed. The nose looks blue and wintry, and wrinkles are brought out as the disease advances, giving an air of premature old age to the patient.

In spite of the loss of strength, he sometimes gets burly and heavy from the growth of soft fat in the cellular tissue; and this increase of weight is a further distress by impeding the exercise of the bodily powers. The nails get friable and crack; the hair is dry and easily falls off; sometimes it quickly turns grey, increasing the aged look before mentioned.

Sometimes the detection of an imperfection of one or other of the senses drives the puzzled invalid to look after his health. He grows deafish without there being any visible cause in the ear to explain deafness, and his aurist finds the usual remedies fail.

Or the sight becomes weak, especially towards evening, and yet his ophthalmic surgeon can find nothing wrong in the eyes.

To the mind of the physiologist, perhaps, the most striking evidence of the defective vital power is in the urine. I have said it is pale and scanty; it is also of lower specific gravity than one would expect from its scantiness. Yet there is not that deposit of lithates which show imperfect assimilation in a healthy person.

Examined under the microscope, it exhibits not infrequently floating crystals of oxalate of lime, and I have heard the irritability of the bladder attributed to the pricking of these sharp crystals. But they are really a great deal too small for that, and, besides, I have found great irritability when they were absent. No; the symptom seems rather due to the deficiency of the normal cause of acidity. For usually the pale urine of these patients is alkaline or neutral, either of which states is sufficient to cause the desire to evacuate the bladder without any diseased state of the urinary organs. The deficiency of urine is not supplemented by any increase in the secretion from the skin as is the case in health. The perspirations are scanty and chilly, and appear to be mere transudations of water instead of being impregnated with the sebaceous secretion as in robust persons.

What I have been endeavouring to depict is the incipient stage of the disease.

If the patient submits his case to the physician, the history seems obscure enough, and indeed consists mainly of negative symptoms. It is not so much that the functions go wrong, as that they do not go on sufficiently. Perhaps sometimes he is told he is 'nervous,' and an effort is made to quiz him into good health. I do not think this quizzing wise or kind. If judicious treatment be employed

I believe the condition to be perfectly amenable to art, and that recovery need not be despaired of if the means of attaining it be taken in good time. But in the majority of instances, unfortunately this does not happen; attention to the general health is postponed till the separate deficiency of some one organ excites alarm as well as discomfort, and enables the ailment to be classified under a more definite name.

This fixing of the disorder in some spot in such a degree as to lead to the diagnosis of the disorganization of that spot, I would designate the second stage.

The failing part is usually one which has been overworked during the early period. If bodily exertion has been persisted in, spite the natural warning to abstain, the heart is very apt to become dilated. In quieter persons some of the arteries become opaque and thickened or dilated, there are throbbings in the head, faintings, threatenings of apoplexy, or perhaps only weakness and irregularity of pulse. If one limb, or certain muscles of one limb, are alone over-exerted as in some peculiar bodily exertions or awkward postures, atrophic paralysis of these often occurs, accompanied by pain in the atrophying parts. This sometimes saves vital viscera by putting a stop to the hurtful employment. Amongst our labouring classes Bright's disease of the kidney is a very usual result. Next to dilated heart it is with hospital patients the commonest local expression of a general degenerative diathesis; whereas in the upper ranks of society Bright's disease is, according to my experience, a primary lesion of the renal tissue, and much less frequently preceded by the injured state of constitution which we are now concerned with. Chronic bronchitis not infrequently appears as the disease advances in middle life. It seems due to the degenerative thickening of the mucous membrane of the air-tubes, and to hardening of the bronchial cartilages.

Atrophic softening of the brain is another local expression of the condition I am describing. It is slow in its progress, often intermittent, less marked in its symptoms, and more likely to be recovered from than where it is a purely local disorder. The conditions thus described are by no means uncommon, and indeed seem on the increase. And while in many cases the effects of climate are not so readily seen where pathological changes have manifested themselves, it is here that we have the greatest promise of these benefits being secured."

T

The cases suitable for the soft, though not damp, winter climate of Rome are chronic bronchitis, phthisis in an early and languid stage, albuminuria without dropsy, some forms of asthma, chronic gastritis, anæmia, and scrofula. Some difference of opinion has existed among physicians regarding the suitability of Rome for persons subject to diarrhœa and dysentery, and an opinion prevails that such cases should not be sent to Italy, and especially to Rome. My own personal experience, and observations in the case of others, leads me to the conclusion that the climate of Italy is peculiarly valuable in many cases both of diarrhœa and dysentery, and especially that variety of the former which is known as *morning* or *rectal diarrhœa*. Fifteen years ago I was invalided from India, after a very severe attack of dysentery. For about two years I tried nearly every remedy, and various climates in England and Scotland, but without deriving any benefit whatever. I was, in short, one of the convalescents who did not continue to convalesce. This was an anxious position, for in health, as in morals, standing still is very rare, and ceasing to make progress is synonymous with falling back. My circulation was so weak, and the difficulty of taking nourishment so great, that, as the months rolled on, I was conscious that ere long some organic change in one or other of the affected organs must show itself and lead to a general and serious break up. With some degree of trembling, I put my house in order and set off for Italy, reaching Florence some time in the beginning of November. Under the homely roof of one of the kindest of landlady's, I was allowed to have very much my own choice in the matter of diet, and *schooled* as I had been in the necessity for carefulness, I carried my English notions into my new Italian home. For several weeks I made but little headway, and, when kind professional and other friends suggested a change in my food as likely to help me, and urged me to follow the example of the Florentines and take a little maccaroni occasionally, with a small wine glass of Chianti, I only shook my head and smiled at the thoughtful and well-meant advice. Gradually, however, and almost without knowing it, I slipped into Italian ways, and, ere the spring had come, I was able to hail returning health, and yet had taken no medicine of any kind. I had simply transferred my home to Florence, had followed the example in matters of diet and exercise of the natives of the place, and felt myself a different man. First, the irregular, and sometimes intermitting, pulse became even in its beat, then stronger and firmer, and soon the heart stroke could be felt with the hand. The muscles regained their power, and, instead of prostration after exertion, there came a healthy feeling of weariness. Alcoholic stimulants were less and less demanded, and the stomach gave little or no trouble. The bowels became strong again, and all traces of dysenteric mischief had passed away, and I was able once more to enter fully into professional work; and to continue it without more than two or three days' break during the lengthened period which it has been my pleasant lot to spend in a country to which I owe so much. What I have said of my experience of Florence is strengthened by a further and more recent experience in Rome. The climate, therefore, in winter, may prove beneficial to the class of cases above enumerated, and to all persons of a lymphatic disposition, with debilitated constitutions, accompanied by languid and feeble circulation, and a tendency to the formation of that lower kind of animal matter which, though it retains the form of the old organ, has little of its vitality, and is known as a degeneration of tissue. When a weak circulation is partly exhibited in neuralgic symptoms, such as constitutional headache, sciatica, intermittent or painless on pressure, without the mucous membranes being involved, the patient may freely enjoy many of the spots in the neighbourhood of the city, as there is not the same need in these cases for shelter and a high temperature.

Spring is the time to enjoy Rome, and no greater mistake is made by visitors than to rush away from it at a time when the country is seen in all its loveliness, and the city itself above its average for healthiness. Of all the months for strangers, April and May are the best, and during the spring and summer, especially if the delightful sea-bathing of the Mediterranean is enjoyed, cases of scrofula, rheumatism, and gout may lay in stores of health sufficient to last them for months or years to come. In the case of patients suffering from atonic or suppressed gout, a protracted residence into the warm summer months is frequently followed by an acute attack which invariably results in much advantage to the patient. In the case of young American and English children, the climate, generally speaking, has the happiest effects, if they are not kept too late in the summer; and more especially are the best results of the climate seen in those having scrofulous or tuberculous tendencies. However, if in these cases symptoms of fever readily show themselves, they must be considered as unsuitable for Rome, and the utmost care requires to be exercised in the matter of children's dress, which is often seen to be insufficient for the requirements of the climate. During the autumn months many of the patients who have passed the summer in the country might make interesting and healthful tours to places too cold for them in winter, and rather too hot to be visited in summer. In some such way as this, the entire year may be profitably and pleasantly spent by those to whom a prolonged residence in the country is necessary to enable them to throw off the tendency to destructive changes which have been described. The only remaining class of travellers which need be referred to can in no sense be termed invalids or patients. There may be some slight degree of nervous exhaustion or brain fag from prolonged or overwork, which calls more for change of scene than change of air. The mind has to be directed into other channels, to receive both rest and occupation in the rich studies of life and character which a tour through Italy affords. To many professional men whose brains are only *weary* from constant wear and tear, no more delightful holiday could be taken than a sojourn in Rome during the month of May. The weather is not too hot to visit the infinite variety of interesting objects within the city, while the *country* is in perfection both as regards climate and beauty of scenery, and with the numerous spots within easy reach of Rome which present to cultured minds the greatest attractions. It is a matter of the utmost surprise that so few scholars and antiquarians take advantage of the opportunity of becoming acquainted with the haunts made famous by Horace, Tacitus, Pliny, and others, and which contain many of the classic ruins of ancient Rome. To the lover of Horace what could be more enjoyable than a day spent exploring the site of his farm and villa, situated as it is in one of the most beautiful valleys of the Sabine country, and of wandering along the high mountain sides which look down upon the clear classic stream of the Licenza, the Digentia of Horace, speeding its way to join the Anio in its course to Rome? Or in visiting Vico Varo, the ancient Varia, perched high upon its rocky foundation, where the five worthy fathers were accustomed to go from Horace's small estate, as burgesses to take part in the settlement of the municipal affairs of the district at the principal town of the valleys? There is no land where there is so much variety to divert the mind from preying on its own thoughts as Italy, and if none of the historical relics interest the traveller, he can scarcely fail to admire their present picturesqueness and the loveliness of the forms and colours by which they are surrounded; while to the social and political observer the specimen of a naturally intellectual and industrious people, long restrained by untoward circumstances and now at length bursting out, for good and for evil, into new life is unique. He desires to live, were it only to see what becomes of them.

The class of patients which should not come to Rome is an important matter, as one frequently sees persons sent here who should have gone elsewhere, and in whom the morbid processes at work were almost certain to become aggravated. All cases to whom excitement of the circulation is injurious should avoid Rome, and therefore persons of apoplectic habit run great risks here. The climate is also prejudicial in some forms of dyspepsia, especially when of a nervous or atonic character; but in these cases attention to a suitable dietary may overcome much of the distress of the illness. All patients having a tendency to congestive inflammation, such as those having weak hearts and imperfect valves, in whom pneumonia is apt to supervene, and cases of tubercular consumption with an excitable circulation and a liability to hæmorrhage, with those who suffer from piles in spite of lessening their daily supply of animal food, and cases of functional diseases of the nervous system, especially hysteria, should not take up their residence in Rome.

To those who do come as invalids it is needless to remind them that they come for the benefit of the climate, to enjoy as much as possible the sunshine, and by spending a considerable portion of their time in the open air be exposed to atmospheric influences likely to prove curative to them in the highest degree. The importance of having an abundance of sunlight, if not always sunshine, cannot be over-rated, while unnecessary exposure at the decline of the day, just before and just after sunset—the hours when the temperature suffers its most sudden and greatest variations must be carefully guarded against, and therefore those afternoon *réunions* in heated rooms, which are so popular in Rome, cannot be too strongly forbidden for those who have come for the benefit of their health, and to whom the observance of certain climatal conditions is of the highest import. These afternoon gatherings are almost a necessity in the purposeless existence led by so many of our countrymen in Italy, but invalids would do well to avoid them. Another matter to be avoided is *self-doctoring*. This practice is rarely without danger anywhere, but it is more than ordinarily dangerous in Rome, and visitors should be particularly careful, especially in the use of quinine. Serious consequences have occurred in Rome from over dosing with this popular drug, and even if such were not the case, much discomfort is often caused and unnecessary alarm felt which would have been avoided had no quinine been taken. There is no drug more used in Rome than quinine, and this is true also of its misuse. During last spring I was asked to visit a gentleman well known in literary circles, residing in the Hotel d'Angleterre. I found him sitting in his snug little room, cowering over the fire, wrapped in a great Scotch plaid, complaining of headache and shivering, and as he said, "All the symptoms of a bad attack of fever coming on." Putting one or two questions to him, I felt satisfied that there was no fever at all in the case, and I learnt that he had been taking during the last twenty-four hours repeated large doses of quinine. He was suffering from Cinchonism; the quinine was stopped and a saline given, with the result that next day he was as well as usual, all his supposed *fever* having disappeared. Cases of this kind are of daily occurrence, and often cause alarm both to the patients and their friends, and it would be well therefore that physicians in other lands should abstain from giving the advice to travellers about to start for Italy to begin a course of the alkaloid as they approach the frontier of the country—an advice which never does any good and often does much harm.

INDEX.

Abetone, The, 4, 21, 243, 249
Accommodation, 193
Acclimatization, 193
Acute diseases in Italy and England, 61
Air, Change of, 1
  ,, Coldness of, 13
  ,, Dampness of, 13
  ,, Dryness of, 10
  ,, Microbes in, 23, 25
  ,, on board steam ships, 8
  ,, Pressure of, 15
  ,, Purity of, 16
  ,, Temperature of, 15
Albano, 215
Alcohol, 196
Amenorrhœa, 14
Andorno, 257
Animal food, 195
Antozone, 35
Appian Way, The, 156
Arricia, 215
Ardenza, The, 220
Arno, Source of, 230
Aqua Albula, 210
  ,, Anio Novus, 164
  ,, ,, Vetus, 158
  ,, Augustan, 163
  ,, Claudia, 164
  ,, Felice, 165
  ,, Hadriana, 164
  ,, Julia, 161
  ,, Marcia, 159
  ,, Paola, 166
  ,, Tepula, 160

Aqua Traiana, 164
  ,, Trevi, 165, 168
  ,, Virgo, 162
  ,, Vergine, 165
Atmosphere, Aqueous vapour of, 11
  ,, Conducting power of, 11
  ,, Functions of, 28
  ,, Humidity of, 26
  ,, Physical properties of, 16
  ,, Saturated, 27
  ,, Stillness of, 34
Australia, 7, 14

Bacillus Malariæ, 139
Baths of Lucca, 233
Biella, 204
Boscolungo, 234
Bologna, 235
Brighton, 14

Camaldoli, 225
Campagna, The, 39, 46, 47, 77, 131
Canada, Climate of, 34
Castel Gandolfo, 215
Cervara, Caves of, 163
Certosa di Pesio, 253
Cervo, Valley of, 204
Chronic disease in Italy, 60
  ,, ,, ,, England, 60
Civita Lavinia, 215
  ,, Vecchia, 207
Climate, 4, 11
  ,, of Rome, 58

INDEX.

Climate of Rome, Physiological effects of, 58
Climates, 17
,, Mountain, Characteristics of, 17
,, ,, Cold dry, 17
,, Physiological effects of, 18
,, Sea, 6, 8
,, ,, Characteristics of, 17
,, Warm and dry, 9
,, ,, inland, 17
,, ,, and moist, 9
,, ,, sea, 17
Colosseum, 194
Curatores Aquarum, 157
Cutigliano, 241

Davos, 5, 19, 30
Dew, 32

Ems, 14
Engadine, 10
Engineers, Early Roman, 153
Eucalyptus trees, 40

Fever, Intermitent, 102
,, Pernicious, 102
,, Roman, 90, 101
,, Remittent, 102
,, Typhoid, 102
Florence, 14
Fogs, 33
Frascati, 214

Gavinana, 237
Ghetto, The, 86
Goitre, 38
,, effects on animals, 39
,, Relation of soil to, 38
Grosetto, 40
Grotto of Monsummano, 219

Halle, 13
Hadrian's Villa 210
Hæmoptysis, 4, 14
Horace, Farm of, 206

Infective Malaria, 125

Janiculum, The, 165

Lago Bracciano, 165
,, Santa Lucia, 164, 185
Lake Albano, 215
,, Nemi, 215
La Paz, 5
,, Spezia, 220
Lavernia, 223, 231
Leghorn, 220
Lerici, Bay of, 42, 221
Ligurian Riviera, The, 221
London, 7, 14
Lucullus, Meadows of, 163, 169

Madeira, 9
Magdeburg, 13
Malaria, Cause of, 132
,, Diffusion of, in Italy, 130
,, Nature of, 132
,, Theories of, 133
,, at sea, 134
,, conveyed by water, 147, 149
,, effects on animals, 40
,, Infective, 125
,, Parasite of, 142
,, ,, Innoculation of animals with, 145
Maloja, The, 5
Mediterranean, The, 42
,, Saltness of, 43
,, High and equable temperature of, 43
Microbes in the air, 24
,, their functions, 24
Mildew, 24
Mineral waters, 201
Mists, 33
Moisture, Absolute, 11, 28
,, Relative, 12, 28
,, of air, 29
,, ,, Clinical significance of, 29
Monte Cavo, 214
Montecatini, 219
Moses, Fountain of, 165
Mould, 136

Naples, 7
,, Bay of, 42

INDEX.

Nervi, 221
Nettuno, 209
Nile, Climate of, 30

Olevano, 213
Orbetello, 40
Orient Line, 7
Organic matters in water, 173
,, ,, Tidy's method of estimating, 173
,, ,, Frankland's method of estimating, 175
Ozone, 15, 35
,, Effects of, 36

Palace of the Cæsars, 45
Palatine, The, 45
Palo, 208
Paris, Typhoid fever in, 103
Pincian Hill, 163
Porto d'Anzio, 208

Quirinal, The, 165
Quito, 5

Rapallo, 221
Riviera, The, 4
,, Eastern, 221
,, Western, 221
Rocca di Papa, 216
Roman Aqueducts, 158
,, Campagna, 39
,, Fever, 90, 100–102
,, ,, Cases of, 110
,, ,, Experincee of, in Florence, 107
,, ,, Nature of, 127
,, ,, Quinine in, 109, 129
,, ,, Symptoms of, 108, 125
,, water, Organic matters in, 172, 173
,, ,, Analysis of, 171
,, wells, 97
Romans, The habits of the, 194
Rome, 14
,, Annual number of visitors to, 94
,, Climate of, 48, 189
,, Closing of wells in, 78

Rome, Cold weather at, 191
,, Height above sea, 46
,, Intramural burying places in, 78
,, Invalids suitable for climate of, 262
,, Latitude of, 45
,, Malarial fever in, 36, 103
,, Number of churches in, 78
,, Population of, 86
,, Prevailing diseases at, 68
,, ,, Winds at, 53
,, Rainfall at, 51
,, Seven Hills of, 46
,, Typhoid fever in, 103
,, Unhealthy dwellings in, 85

Salone, Valley of, 163
San Marcello, 240
San Giovanni Hospital, 64
,, ,, Malarial fevers in, 64
,, ,, Acute diseases of lungs in, 64
St. Moritz, 5, 19, 30
Sacro Eremo, 225, 229
Santa Margherita, 221
Sanctuarii, The, 204
Santo Spirito Hospital, 62
,, ,, Malarial fevers in, 63
,, ,, Acute diseases of lungs in, 63
Scrofula, 14
Sea air, Bromine in, 20
,, ,, Iodine in, 20
Sestri, 221
Settling Reservoirs, 155
Siberia, Climate of, 34
Sleeplessness, 196
Soil, Chemical nature of, 37
,, Mineralogical nature of, 37
,, Geological formation of, 37
Stagnant water, Pernicious influence of, 79
Subcontinued typhoid, 105
Subiaco, 206, 211
Sublaqueum, 213
Subsoil water, 41
Suburbs of Rome, 198

INDEX.

Sun, Influence of, on dry air, 31
,, ,, ,, moist air, 31
Sunrise, 199
Sunset, 133, 199

Tiber, The, 46
,, Source of, 230
Tivoli, 211
Tramontana, The, 2
Trastevere, 165
Tuscan Maremma, The, 39
Tusculum, 214

Typhoid fever in Rome, 72
,, ,, Paris, 72
,, Subcontinued, 103

Vallombrosa, 223
Via Reggio, 220
Via Sublacensis, 185, 211
,, Valeria, 185, 211
Visitors, Imprudence of, 194

Winds, 53

October, 1885.

SELECTED LIST OF

NEW AND RECENT WORKS

PUBLISHED BY

H. K. LEWIS,

136 GOWER STREET, LONDON, W.C.

** *For full list of works in Medicine and Surgery published by H. K. Lewis see Complete Catalogue sent post free on application.*

FREDERICK T. ROBERTS, M.D., B.SC., F.R.C.P.

Examiner in Medicine at the Royal College of Surgeons; Professor of Therapeutics in University College; Physician to University College Hospital; Physician to the Brompton Consumption Hospital, &c.

A HANDBOOK OF THE THEORY AND PRACTICE OF MEDICINE. Sixth Edition, with Illustrations, in one volume of over 1000 pages, large 8vo, 21s. [*Just published.*

NOTICES OF THE PRESS.

" The amount of information in this book, is, for its size, enormous. . . . The book seems to be thoroughly trustworthy, and those who read it may be sure that the views put before them are not the fanciful notions of the few, but the well-considered and generally adopted ideas of our leading scientific practitioners." " Abounds in information supplied in a thoroughly systematic manner."—*Lancet.*

" The various subjects have been treated in a complete and masterly manner. . . . . We heartily commend this handbook, not only to gentlemen preparing for the medical profession, but to those who have finished their professional education; as this work contains, in a brief and concise shape, all that the busy practitioner needs to know to enable him to carry on his practice with comfort to himself and with advantage to his patients."—*British Medical Journal.*

" We have already on more than one occasion expressed a high opinion as to the merits of this work. . . . . From our experience of the ' Handbook,' we believe that it will always be popular amongst medical students, and that it is sufficiently classical to deserve a place on the bookshelves of every physician. . . . . We heartily commend it as a reliable guide not less to the practical than to the theoretical study of medicine."—*Dublin Journal of Medical Science.*

BY THE SAME AUTHOR.

NOTES ON MATERIA MEDICA AND PHARMACY.
Fcap. 8vo, 7s. 6d. [*Now ready.*

NOTICES OF THE PRESS.

" Will soon be a favourite handbook for students."—*Medical Chronicle.*

"Well adapted to the requirements of students preparing for examination." *Lancet.*

"An admirably constructed recapitulation of facts necessary to be recollected."—*Pharmaceutical Journal.*

"As a handbook to Materia Medica and Pharmacy it is eminently the one most suited for examination purposes."—*Student's Journal.*

JOHN R. WARDELL, M.D., F.R.C.P.
Late Consulting Physician to Tunbridge Wells General Hospital.

CONTRIBUTIONS TO PATHOLOGY AND THE PRACTICE OF MEDICINE. Medium 8vo, 21s.

GENERAL CONTENTS.

Hypertrophy of the Heart—Diseases of the Spleen—Diseases of the Pancreas—Enteralgia—Peritonitis—Enteritis—Ulceration of the Bowels—Carcinoma of the Bowels—Fatal Obstruction of the Bowels caused by a Band of Lymph—Acute Peritonitis and Displacement of the Cæcum—Pelvic Cellulitis—Apoplexy—Pleuritic, Serous, and Purulent Effusions—Chronic Ulcer of the Stomach—Carcinoma of the Liver—Typhoid or Enteric Fever—Relapsing Fever—Subclavian Aneurism—Aneurism of the Left Ventricle—Diffuse Aneurism of the Abdominal Aorta—Obesity—Hydronephrosis—Hæmatocele connected with the Left Kidney—Uræmia—Chronic Ulceration of the Urinary Bladder, with Hæmorrhage—Exfoliation of the Bladder—Small Fatty Growths obstructing the Cystic and Common Ducts—Chorea—Tubercular Meningitis—Myeloid Sarcoma Tumour of the Brain—Syphilitic Tumour at the Base of the Brain—Syphilitic Hemiplegia—Scorbutus—Erythema Circinatum—Lupus Erythematosus treated by Lemon-Juice—Puerperal Convulsions—Enlargement of the Spleen in Leucocythæmia—Spasmus Glottidis—Croup—Chronic Glossitis—Tæniæ—Infanticide—Suspected Poisoning—Poisoning by Laudanum—Lead Palsy- Poisoning by Sulphuric Acid—Poisoning by Burnett's Disinfecting Fluid—A Thorn in the Flesh—Advanced and Present Medicine.

C. H. RALFE, M.A., M.D. CANTAB., F.R.C.P. LOND.

Assistant Physician to the London Hospital; late Senior Physician to the Seamen's Hospital, Greenwich.

A PRACTICAL TREATISE OF DISEASES OF THE KIDNEYS AND URINARY DERANGEMENTS. With Illustrations, crown 8vo, 10s. 6d. *[Now ready.* Lewis's Practical Series.]

GENERAL CONTENTS.

General Symptomatology of Kidney Disease—Clinical Examination of Urine—Diffuse Inflammation of the Kidney—Suppurative Inflammation of the Kidney, etc.—Degenerations and Infiltrations of the Kidney—New Growths in the Kidney—Parasites in the Kidney—Abnormalities of the Kidney—Variations in the Amount of Urine—Stone and Gravel—Functional Albuminuria, Peptonuria and Hæmoglobinuria—Quantitative estimation of Urea, etc.—Diet Table.

HENRY R. SWANZY, A.M., M.B., F.R.C.S.I.

Examiner in Ophthalmic Surgery at the Royal College of Surgeons, Ireland; Surgeon to the National Eye and Ear Infirmary, Dublin; Ophthalmic Surgeon to the Adelaide Hospital, Dublin; Formerly Assistant to the late Professor A. von Graefe, Berlin.

A HANDBOOK OF DISEASES OF THE EYE AND THEIR TREATMENT. Illustrated with Wood Engravings, Colour Tests, etc., large post 8vo, 10s. 6d.

NOTICES OF THE PRESS.

" We have great pleasure in recommending this work to all students and practitioners who desire to acquire such a knowledge of the defects and diseases of the eye as will render them competent to recognise and undertake the treatment of any ordinary case which may present itself in practice."—*Lancet.*

"We must admit that this (textbook) justifies its presence by its admirable type illustrations and dress, by its clear wording, and above all by the vast amount of varied matter which it embraces within the relatively small compass of some 400 pages."—*British Medical Journal.*

" This is an excellent textbook, written by a surgeon of large experience and a thorough knowledge of the literature of his subject."— *The Edinburgh Medical Journal.*

" This handbook is in our opinion an admirable one. . . . There is throughout a clearness of detail, especially in regard to treatment, therapeutic as well as operative, which denotes the surgeon of wide experience, and which will certainly make the book a favourite. . . . The book is capitally illustrated and well printed."— *Ophthalmic Review.*

EDGAR M. CROOKSHANK, M.B. LOND.

BACTERIOLOGY : PRACTICAL, SYSTEMATIC, AND DESCRIPTIVE. An introduction to the study of Bacteria, based upon the most recent methods employed by the school of Koch. With Appendix, including a description of Yeast and Mould Fungi, and the methods of examination of Air, Soil and Water. With Coloured Illustrations from Original Drawings and numerous Woodcuts. [*In the press.*

GENERAL CONTENTS.

PART I. Apparatus, Material, and Reagents employed in a Bacteriological Laboratory—Microscopical Examination of Bacteria, in Liquids, Cultivations on Solid Media, and Tissues—Preparation and Staining of Tissue Sections—Preparation of Nutrient Media and Methods of Cultivation—Experiments upon the Living Animal—Examination of Experimental Animals after Death.

PART II. Classification and Description of Bacteria.

BERKELEY HILL, M.B. LOND., F.R.C.S.
Professor of Clinical Surgery in University College; Surgeon to University College Hospital, and to the Lock Hospital.

THE ESSENTIALS OF BANDAGING. For Managing Fractures and Dislocations; for administering Ether and Chloroform ; and for using other Surgical Apparatus. Fifth Edition, revised and much enlarged, with Illustrations, fcap. 8vo, 5s.

BERKELEY HILL, M.B. LOND., F.R.C.S.
Professor of Clinical Surgery in University College; Surgeon to University College Hospital, and to the Lock Hospital.

AND

ARTHUR COOPER, L.R.C.P., M.R.C.S.
Surgeon to the Westminster General Dispensary, &c.

I.

SYPHILIS AND LOCAL CONTAGIOUS DISORDERS. Second Edition, entirely re-written, royal 8vo, 18s.

II.

THE STUDENT'S MANUAL OF VENEREAL DISEASES. Being a Concise Description of those Affections and of their Treatment. Third Edition, post 8vo, 2s. 6d.

W. H. O. SANKEY, M.D. LOND., F.R.C.P.

Late Lecturer on Mental Diseases, University College, and School of Medicine, London; Formerly Medical Superintendent (Female Department) of Hanwell Asylum; President of Medico-Psychological Society, &c.

LECTURES ON MENTAL DISEASE. Second Edition, with coloured plates, 8vo, 12s. 6d.

A. DE WATTEVILLE, M.A., M.D., B.SC., M.R.C.S.

Physician in Charge of the Electro-therapeutical Department of St. Mary's Hospital.

A PRACTICAL INTRODUCTION TO MEDICAL ELECTRICITY. Second Edition, re-written and enlarged, copiously Illustrated, 8vo, 9s.

EDWARD WOAKES, M.D.

Senior Aural Surgeon and Lecturer on Aural Surgery at the London Hospital; Senior Surgeon to the Hospital for Diseases of the Throat.

ON DEAFNESS, GIDDINESS, AND NOISES IN THE HEAD.

PART I.—POST-NASAL CATARRH, AND DISEASES OF THE NOSE CAUSING DEAFNESS. With Illustrations, crown 8vo, 6s. 6d.

PART II.—ON DEAFNESS, GIDDINESS, AND NOISES IN THE HEAD. Third Edition, with Illustrations, crown 8vo. [*In preparation.*

E. CRESSWELL BABER, M.B., L.R.C.P., M.R.C.S.

Hon. Surgeon to the Brighton Hove and Sussex Throat and Ear Dispensary.

ON THE EXAMINATION OF THE NOSE. Large post 8vo. [*In the press.*

G. GRANVILLE BANTOCK, M.D., F.R.C.S. EDIN.
Surgeon to the Samaritan Free Hospital for Women and Children.

ON THE USE AND ABUSE OF PESSARIES. With Illustrations, Second Edition, 8vo, 5s.

FANCOURT BARNES, M.D., M.R.C.P.
Physician to the Chelsea Hospital; Obstetric Physician to the Great Northern Hospital, &c.

A GERMAN-ENGLISH DICTIONARY OF WORDS AND TERMS USED IN MEDICINE AND ITS COGNATE SCIENCES. Square 12mo, Roxburgh binding, 9s.

ROBERTS BARTHOLOW, M.A., M.D., LL.D.
Professor of Materia Medica and Therapeutics in the Jefferson Medical College of Philadelphia, etc.

I.

A TREATISE ON THE PRACTICE OF MEDICINE FOR THE USE OF STUDENTS AND PRACTITIONERS. With Illustrations, 5th Edition, large 8vo, 21s.
[*Just published*.

II.

A PRACTICAL TREATISE ON MATERIA MEDICA AND THERAPEUTICS. Fifth Edition, Revised and Enlarged, 8vo, 18s. [*Now ready*.

GEO. M. BEARD, A.M., M.D.
Fellow of the New York Academy of Medicine.

AND

A. D. ROCKWELL, A.M., M.D.
Fellow of the New York Academy of Medicine.

A PRACTICAL TREATISE ON THE MEDICAL AND SURGICAL USES OF ELECTRICITY; including Localized and General Faradization; Localized and Central Galvanization; Electrolysis and Galvano-Cautery. Fourth Edit. With nearly 200 Illustrations, roy. 8vo, 28s.

A. HUGHES BENNETT, M.D.

Member of the Royal College of Physicians of London; Physician to the Hospital for Epilepsy and Paralysis, Regent's Park; and Assistant Physician to the Westminster Hospital.

I.

A PRACTICAL TREATISE ON ELECTRO-DIAGNOSIS IN DISEASES OF THE NERVOUS SYSTEM. With Illustrations, 8vo, 8s. 6d.

II.

ILLUSTRATIONS OF THE SUPERFICIAL NERVES AND MUSCLES, WITH THEIR MOTOR POINTS, A knowledge of which is essential in the art of Electro-Diagnosis. (Extracted from the above). 8vo, paper cover 1s. 6d., cloth 2s.

ALFRED H. CARTER, M.D. LOND.

Member of the Royal College of Physicians; Physician to the Queen's Hospital, Birmingham; Examiner in Medicine for the University of Aberdeen, &c.

ELEMENTS OF PRACTICAL MEDICINE. Third Edition, crown 8vo, 9s.

P. CAZEAUX.

Adjunct Professor in the Faculty of Medicine of Paris, &c.

AND

S. TARNIER.

Professor of Obstetrics and Diseases of Women and Children in the Faculty of Medicine of Paris.

OBSTETRICS: THE THEORY AND PRACTICE; including the Diseases of Pregnancy and Parturition, Obstetrical Operations, &c. Seventh Edition, edited and revised by ROBERT J. HESS, M.D., with twelve full-page plates, five being coloured, and 165 wood-engravings, 1081 pages, royal 8vo, 35s.

W. H. CORFIELD, M.A., M.D. OXON.

Professor of Hygiene and Public Health in University College, London.

DWELLING HOUSES: their Sanitary Construction and Arrangements. Second Edition, with Illustrations, crown 8vo, 3s. 6d.

EDWARD COTTERELL, M.R.C.S. ENG., L.R.C.P. LOND.

Late House Surgeon, University College Hospital; Atkinson Morley Surgical Scholar, University College, London, etc. etc.

ON SOME COMMON INJURIES TO LIMBS: their Treatment and After-Treatment including Bone-Setting (so-called). Imp. 16mo, with Illustrations, 3s. 6d.

J. MILNER FOTHERGILL, M.D.

Member of the Royal College of Physicians of London; Physician to the City of London Hospital for Diseases of the Chest, Victoria Park, &c.

I.

THE HEART AND ITS DISEASES, WITH THEIR TREATMENT; INCLUDING THE GOUTY HEART. Second Edition, entirely re-written, copiously illustrated with woodcuts and lithographic plates. 8vo, 16s.

II.

INDIGESTION, BILIOUSNESS, AND GOUT IN ITS PROTEAN ASPECTS.

PART I.—INDIGESTION AND BILIOUSNESS.
Post 8vo, 7s 6d.

PART II.—GOUT IN ITS PROTEAN ASPECTS.
Post 8vo, 7s. 6d.

HENEAGE GIBBES, M.D.

Lecturer on Physiology and Histology in the Medical School of Westminster Hospital; late Curator of the Anatomical Museum at King's College.

PRACTICAL HISTOLOGY AND PATHOLOGY. Third Edition, revised and enlarged, crown 8vo, 6s.

[*Just ready.*

J. B. GRESSWELL, M.R.C.V.S.

Provincial Veterinary Surgeon to the Royal Agricultural Society.

VETERINARY PHARMACOLOGY AND THERAPEUTICS. Fcap. 8vo, 5s.

WILLIAM A. HAMMOND, M.D.
Professor of Mental and Nervous Diseases in the Medical Department of the University of the City of New York.

I.

A TREATISE ON THE DISEASES OF THE NERVOUS SYSTEM. Seventh Edition, with 112 Illustrations, large 8vo, 25s.

II.

A TREATISE ON INSANITY. Large 8vo, 25s.

GEORGE LINDSAY JOHNSON, M.A., M.B., B.C. CANTAB.
Clinical Assistant, late House Surgeon and Chloroformist, Royal Westminster Ophthalmic Hospital.

A NEW METHOD OF TREATING CHRONIC GLAUCOMA: Based on Recent Researches into its Pathology. With Illustrations and Coloured Frontispiece, demy 8vo, 3s. 6d.

RUSTOMJEE NASERWANJEE KHORY, M.D. BRUX., M.R.C.P.

THE PRINCIPLES AND PRACTICE OF MEDICINE. Second Edition, revised and much enlarged, 2 vols., large 8vo, 28s.

J. WICKHAM LEGG, F.R.C.P.
Assistant Physician to Saint Bartholomew's Hospital, and Lecturer on Pathological Anatomy in the Medical School.

I.

ON THE BILE, JAUNDICE, AND BILIOUS DISEASES. With Illustrations in chromo-lithography, 719 pages, roy. 8vo, 25s.

II.

A GUIDE TO THE EXAMINATION OF THE URINE; intended chiefly for Clinical Clerks and Students. Sixth Edition, revised and enlarged, with additional Illustrations, fcap. 8vo, 2s 6d.

LEWIS'S PRACTICAL SERIES.

Under this title Mr. Lewis is publishing a complete series of Monographs embracing the various branches of Medicine and Surgery.

The volumes, written by well-known Hospital Physicians and Surgeons recognised as authorities in the subjects of which they treat, are in active preparation. The works are intended to be of a thoroughly Practical nature, calculated to meet the requirements of the general Practitioner, and to present the most recent information in a compact and readable form; the volumes will be handsomely got up, issued at low prices, varying with the size of the works.

THE FOLLOWING ARE NOW READY.

BODILY DEFORMITIES AND THEIR TREATMENT: A Handbook of Practical Orthopædics. By H. A. REEVES, F.R.C.S. Ed., Senior Assistant Surgeon and Teacher of Practical Surgery at the London Hospital, Surgeon to the Royal Orthopædic Hospital, etc. With numerous Illustrations, crown 8vo, 8s. 6d.

DENTAL SURGERY FOR GENERAL PRACTITIONERS AND STUDENTS OF MEDICINE. By ASHLEY W. BARRETT, M.B. Lond., M.R.C.S., L.D.S., Dental Surgeon to, and Lecturer on Dental Surgery and Pathology in the Medical School of, the London Hospital. With Illustrations, crown 8vo, 3s.

A PRACTICAL TREATISE ON DISEASES OF THE KID- NEYS AND URINARY DERANGEMENTS. By C. H. RALFE, M.D. Cantab., F.R.C.P. Lond., Assistant Physician to the London Hospital, late Senior Physician to the Seamen's Hospital, Greenwich. With Illustrations, crown 8vo, 10s. 6d. *[Now ready.*

*** Prospectus of the Series, with Specimen page, etc., post free on application.

LEWIS'S POCKET MEDICAL VOCABULARY.
[In the press.

WILLIAM THOMPSON LUSK, A.M., M.D.
Professor of Obstetrics and Diseases of Women in the Bellevue Hospital Medical College, &c.

THE SCIENCE AND ART OF MIDWIFERY. Second Edition, with numerous Illustrations, 8vo, 18s.

JOHN MACPHERSON, M.D.
Inspector-General of Hospitals H.M. Bengal Army (Retired).
Author of "Cholera in its Home," &c.

ANNALS OF CHOLERA FROM THE EARLIEST PERIODS TO THE YEAR 1817. With a map. Demy 8vo, 7s. 6d.

A. COWLEY MALLEY, B.A., M.B., B.CH. T.C.D.

PHOTO-MICROGRAPHY; including a description of the Wet Collodion and Gelatino-Bromide Processes, together with the best methods of mounting and preparing Microscopic Objects for Photo-Micrography. Second Edition, with Illustrations and Photographs, crown 8vo, 7s. 6d.

PATRICK MANSON, M.D., C.M.
Amoy, China.

THE FILARIA SANGUINIS HOMINIS AND CERTAIN NEW FORMS OF PARASITIC DISEASE IN INDIA, CHINA, AND WARM COUNTRIES. Illustrated with Plates, Woodcuts, and Charts. Demy 8vo, 10s. 6d.

S. E. MAUNSELL, L.R.C.S.I.
Surgeon-Major, Medical Staff.

NOTES OF MEDICAL EXPERIENCES IN INDIA PRINCIPALLY WITH REFERENCE TO DISEASES OF THE EYE. With Map, post 8vo, 3s. 6d.

J. F. MEIGS, M.D.
Consulting Physician to the Children's Hospital, Philadelphia.

AND

W. PEPPER, M.D.
Lecturer on Clinical Medicine in the University of Pennsylvania.

A PRACTICAL TREATISE ON THE DISEASES OF CHILDREN. Seventh Edition, revised and enlarged roy. 8vo, 28s.

WILLIAM MARTINDALE, F.C.S.
Late Examiner of the Pharmaceutical Society, and late Teacher of Pharmacy and Demonstrator of Materia Medica at University College.

AND

W. WYNN WESTCOTT, M.B. LOND.
Deputy Coroner for Central Middlesex.

THE EXTRA PHARMACOPŒIA of Unofficial Drugs and Chemical and Pharmaceutical Preparations. With References to their Use abstracted from the Medical Journals, and a Therapeutic Index of Diseases and Symptoms. Fourth Edition, revised with numerous additions, limp roan, med. 24mo. [*In the press.*

WM. JULIUS MICKLE, M.D., M.R.C.P.
Member of the Medico-Psychological Association of Great Britain and Ireland; Member of the Clinical Society, London; Medical Superintendent, Grove Hall Asylum, London.

GENERAL PARALYSIS OF THE INSANE. 8vo, 10s.

A. STANFORD MORTON, M.B., F.R.C.S. ED.
Senior Assistant Surgeon, Royal South London Ophthalmic Hospital.

REFRACTION OF THE EYE: Its Diagnosis, and the Correction of its Errors, with Chapter on Keratoscopy. Second Edition. Small 8vo, 2s. 6d.

WILLIAM MURRELL, M.D., F.R.C.P.
Lecturer on Materia Medica and Therapeutics at Westminster Hospital; Examiner in Materia Medica and Therapeutics in the University of Edinburgh, and to the Royal College of Physicians, London.

WHAT TO DO IN CASES OF POISONING. Fourth Edition, revised and enlarged, royal 32mo, 3s. 6d.

DR. FELIX VON NIEMEYER.
Late Professor of Pathology and Therapeutics; Director of the Medical Clinic of the University of Tübingen.

A TEXT-BOOK OF PRACTICAL MEDICINE, WITH PARTICULAR REFERENCE TO PHYSIOLOGY AND PATHOLOGICAL ANATOMY. Translated from the Eighth German Edition, by special permission of the Author, by GEORGE H. HUMPHREY, M.D., and CHARLES E. HACKLEY, M.D. Revised Edition, 2 vols., large 8vo, 36s.

G. OLIVER, M.D., M.R.C.P.

I.

ON BEDSIDE URINE TESTING: a Clinical Guide the Observation of Urine in the course of Work. Thi Edition, considerably enlarged, fcap. 8vo, 3s. 6d. [*Just publishe*

II.

THE HARROGATE WATERS: Data Chemical and Therapeutical, with notes on the Climate of Harrogate. Addressed to the Medical Profession. Crown 8vo, with Map of the Wells, 3s. 6d.

R. W. PARKER.
Surgeon to the East London Hospital for Women and Children and to the Grosvenor Hospital for Women and Children.

TRACHEOTOMY IN LARYNGEAL DIPHTHERIA; AFTER TREATMENT AND COMPLICATIONS. Second Edition, with Illustrations, 8vo, 5s.

G. V. POORE, M.D., F.R.C.P.
Professor of Medical Jurisprudence, University College; Assistant Physician and Physician in charge of the Throat Department of University College Hospital.

LECTURES ON THE PHYSICAL EXAMINATION OF THE MOUTH AND THROAT. With an appendix of Cases. 8vo, 3s. 6d.

R. DOUGLAS POWELL, M.D., F.R.C.P., M.R.C.S.
Physician to the Hospital for Consumption and Diseases of the Chest at Brompton, Physician to the Middlesex Hospital.

DISEASES OF THE LUNGS AND PLEURÆ. Third Edition, re-written and enlarged, with Illustrations, 8vo. [*In the press.*

SYDNEY RINGER, M.D.,
Professor of the Principles and Practice of Medicine in University College; Physician to, and Professor of Clinical Medicine in, University College Hospital.

A HANDBOOK OF THERAPEUTICS. Eleventh Edition, revised, 8vo. [*In preparation.*

A. R. ROBINSON, M.B., L.R.C.P. & L.R.C.S. EDIN.
Professor of Dermatology at the New York Polyclinic.

A MANUAL OF DERMATOLOGY. With 88 Illustrations, large 8vo, 21s.

D. B. ST. JOHN ROOSA, M.A., M.D.
Professor of Diseases of the Eye and Ear in the University of the City of New York; Surgeon to the Manhattan Eye and Ear Hospital; Consulting Surgeon to the Brooklyn Eye and Ear Hospital, &c., &c.

A PRACTICAL TREATISE ON THE DISEASES OF THE EAR, including the Anatomy of the Organ. Sixth Edition, Illustrated by wood engravings and chromo-lithographs, large 8vo, 25s.

ROBSON ROOSE, M.D., F.R.C.P. EDIN.

GOUT, AND ITS RELATIONS TO DISEASES OF THE LIVER AND KIDNEYS. Crown 8vo, 3s. 6d.

ALDER SMITH, M.B. LOND., F.R.C.S.
Resident Medical Officer, Christ's Hospital, London.

RINGWORM: ITS DIAGNOSIS AND TREATMENT. Third Edition, rewritten and enlarged, with Illustrations, fcap. 8vo, 5s. 6d.

J. LEWIS SMITH, M.D.
Physician to the New York Infants' Hospital; Clinical Lecturer on Diseases of Children in Bellevue Hospital Medical College.

A TREATISE ON THE DISEASES OF INFANCY AND CHILDHOOD. Fifth Edition, with Illustrations, large 8vo, 21s.

FRANCIS W. SMITH, M.B., B.S.

THE SALINE WATERS OF LEAMINGTON: Chemically, Therapeutically, and Clinically Considered; with Observations on the Climate of Leamington. Second Edition, with Illustrations, crown 8vo, 1s. *nett*.

EDWARD T. TIBBITS, M.D. LOND.
Physician to the Bradford Infirmary and to the Bradford Fever Hospital.

MEDICAL FASHIONS IN THE NINETEENTH CENTURY: including a sketch of Bacterio-Mania and the Battle of the Bacilli. Crown 8vo, 2s. 6d.

FREDERICK TREVES, F.R.C.S.
Hunterian Professor at the Royal College of Surgeons of England; Surgeon to, and Lecturer on Anatomy at, the London Hospital.

THE ANATOMY OF THE INTESTINAL CANAL AND PERITONEUM IN MAN. Hunterian Lectures, 1885. 4to, 2s. 6d.

D. HACK TUKE, LL.D., F.R.C.P.

THE INSANE IN THE UNITED STATES AND CANADA. 8vo, 7s. 6d.

A. DUNBAR WALKER, M.D., C.M.

THE PARENTS' MEDICAL NOTE BOOK. Oblong post 8vo, cloth, 1s. 6d.

W. SPENCER WATSON, F.R.C.S., M.B.
Surgeon to the Great Northern Hospital; Surgeon to the Royal South London Ophthalmic Hospital.

DISEASES OF THE NOSE AND ITS ACCESSORY CAVITIES. Profusely Illustrated, demy 8vo, 18s.

FRANCIS WELCH, F.R.C.S.
Surgeon-Major, A.M.D.

ENTERIC FEVER: its Prevalence and Modifications; Etiology; Pathology and Treatment; as illustrated by Army Data at Home and Abroad. Demy 8vo, 5s. 6d.

W. WYNN WESTCOTT, M.B. LOND.
Deputy Coroner for Central Middlesex.

SUICIDE: its History, Literature, Jurisprudence, Causation and Prevention. Crown 8vo, 6s.

E. T. WILSON, B.M. OXON., F.R.C.P. LOND.
Physician to the Cheltenham General Hospital and Dispensary.

DISINFECTANTS AND HOW TO USE THEM. In Packets of one doz. price 1s.

CLINICAL CHARTS FOR TEMPERATURE OBSERVATIONS, ETC. Arranged by W. RIGDEN, M.R.C.S. Price 7s. per 100, or 1s. per doz.

Each Chart is arranged for four weeks, and is ruled at the back for making notes of cases; they are convenient in size, and are suitable both for hospital and private practice.

PERIODICAL WORKS PUBLISHED BY H. K. LEWIS.

THE NEW SYDENHAM SOCIETY'S PUBLICATIONS. Annual Subscription, One Guinea.
(Report of the Society, with Complete List of Works and other information, gratis on application).

THE NEW YORK MEDICAL JOURNAL. A Weekly Review of Medicine. Annual Subscription, One Guinea, post free.

ARCHIVES OF PEDIATRICS. A Monthly Journal, devoted to the Diseases of Infants and Children. Annual Subscription, 12s. 6d., post free.

MEDICAL BULLETIN. A Monthly Journal of Medicine and Surgery. Edited by Dr. J. V. Shoemaker. Annual Subscription, 5s.

THE THERAPEUTIC GAZETTE. A Monthly Journal, devoted to the Science of Pharmacology, and to the introduction of New Therapeutic Agents. Edited by Drs. H. C. Wood and R. M. Smith. Annual Subscription, 10s., post free.

THE GLASGOW MEDICAL JOURNAL. Published Monthly. Annual Subscription, 20s., post free. Single numbers, 2s. each.

LIVERPOOL MEDICO-CHIRURGICAL JOURNAL, including the Proceedings of the Liverpool Medical Institution. Published twice yearly, 3s. 6d. each number.

THE PROVINCIAL MEDICAL JOURNAL. Edited by Thomas M. Dolan, M.D. Annual Subscription, 7s. 6d., post free.

TRANSACTIONS OF THE COLLEGE OF PHYSICIANS OF PHILADELPHIA. Volumes I. to VI., now ready, 8vo, 10s. 6d. each.

THE INDIAN MEDICAL JOURNAL. A Journal of Medical and Sanitary Science specially devoted to the Interests of the Medical Services. Annual Subscription, 24s., post free.

*** Mr. Lewis has transactions with the leading publishing firms in America for the sale of his publications in that country. Arrangements are made in the interests of Authors either for sending a number of copies of their works to the United States, or having them reprinted there, as may be most advantageous.

Mr. Lewis's publications can be procured of any bookseller in any part of the world.

Complete Catalogue of Publications post free on application.

Printed by H. K. Lewis, Gower Street, London, W.C.